Y0-EKS-304

Refreshing! Revitalizing! Rejuvenating!

Everything you need to make your complexion come alive is at your fingertips in

THE HOME GUIDE TO NATURAL BEAUTY CARE

Discover the ancient cosmetic secrets of fruits and vegetables, oils and herbs—and combat the skin's worst enemies such as dehydration, sun exposure, allergies and skin sensitivities. Here are easy, at-home recipes for 100% natural skin care treatments—from cleansers and toners to moisturizers and refreshers. Give your skin a dazzling, youthful glow—and become a gourmet of natural skin care!

Most Berkley Books are available at special quantity discounts for bulk purchases for sales promotions, premiums, fund-raising or educational use. Special books, or book excerpts, can also be created to fit specific needs.

For details, write or telephone Special Markets, The Berkley Publishing Group, 200 Madison Avenue, New York, New York 10016; (212) 951-8891

THE HOME GUIDE TO NATURAL BEAUTY CARE

JULIA BUSCH

Previously published as
TREAT YOUR FACE LIKE A SALAD

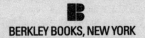

BERKLEY BOOKS, NEW YORK

If you purchased this book without a cover, you should be aware that this book is stolen property. It was reported as "unsold and destroyed" to the publisher, and neither the author nor the publisher has received any payment for this "stripped book."

Originally published under the title *Treat Your Face Like a Salad.*

The purpose of this book is to educate and entertain. It is not the intent of this book to serve in any way whatsoever as a program for self-treatment of medical problems. Medical problems should be brought to the attention of the reader's physician. Any application of the concepts and/or information contained in this book is done solely at the risk and the discretion of the reader.

THE HOME GUIDE TO NATURAL BEAUTY CARE

A Berkley Book / published by arrangement with
Anti-Aging Press, Inc.

PRINTING HISTORY
Anti-Aging Press edition published 1993
Berkley edition / February 1995

All rights reserved.
Copyright © 1993 by Julia M. Busch.
Illustrations copyright © 1993 by Julia M. Busch.
This book may not be reproduced in whole or in part,
by mimeograph or any other means, without permission.
For information address: Anti-Aging Press, Inc.,
P.O. Box 1489, Coral Gables, Florida 33114.

ISBN: 0-425-14573-5

BERKLEY®
Berkley Books are published by The Berkley Publishing Group,
200 Madison Avenue, New York, New York 10016.
BERKLEY and the "B" design
are trademarks belonging to Berkley Publishing Corporation.

PRINTED IN THE UNITED STATES OF AMERICA

10 9 8 7 6 5 4 3 2 1

TO
THE FABU-LISHOUS FACES
I DEARLY LOVE!

ACKNOWLEDGMENTS

Thank you:

Lynn Whittick, enthusiastic editing!

ASPA, The American Association for Phytotherapy and Aromatherapy International.

Aromatherapists, herbalists and nutritionists, who have generously published a wealth of information from which I have heavily drawn.

Wally Engelhard and "eagle-eye" Shirlee Dreyer of Engelhard Printing, Miami, and Joan Mangrum, Braun-Brumfield.

Gary Winer, computer, technical advice and support.

Ben Woodworth, "cover" consults.

And, as ever, "Mom," Hollye—and Steven, who always anxiously awaits the "next" book.

It was my pleasure.

CONTENTS

THE "FABU-LISHOUS" FACE

Ever fight back an overwhelming urge to taste a succulent cheek? How about those pinchable, dewy, round, rosies—deliciously edible faces that could do with just a little nibbling—clean, clear, crisp, luscious, radiant skin that sets your senses tingling. Well, ladies and gentlemen, dazzling, wrinkle-and-blemish-free-skin can be yours at any age. With the proper care, blemishes can fade, wrinkles diminish (or downright disappear), muscles tone, and skin glow all over—all without commercial cosmetics, in fact, better without commercial cosmetics.

Why? Simply because of the ingredients. You know what you are getting. You know the fixin's are fresh, potent and preservative free. Even the best natural cosmetics contain preservatives and lose vitality sitting on the shelf, and a papaya fresh from the market will "clarify" your skin without acetone, the expensive department store exfoliant that also removes nail polish.

End the cosmetics confusion. Forget all the options: "Should I tissue off, rub or rinse, freshen, astringe or tone?" Ignore all the hype!

Good skin care is very simple. Beautiful skin has existed for centuries, ask Cleopatra and the ladies of the French court. Just treat your face like a salad! Clean it. Crisp it. Mist it. Press it. Dress it with nutrient-replenishing, skin-tightening, blemish-fading, wrinkle-erasing, acne-clearing natural at-home recipes and gourmet hints for a fabu-lishous face.

I.
SUCCULENT, SEDUCTIVE SKIN:
THE BASICS

"RIPE READY MELONS!"

What do a ripe, ready melon, an engorged grape, a prime purple plum and a crisp crunchy apple all have in common? Juice! Without juice all the salivating seduction of fruit turns to raisins and prunes. Not much of a fruit salad. And limp lettuce languishing in the larder is part of tomorrow's trash. Without "juice," skin doesn't fare any better. So, for succulent, seductive skin, water is your most important asset.

To maintain your moisture balance you need to know only two things—hydrate your skin from the inside and hydrate from the outside. In other words, drink enough fluids to plump your inner skin and keep your outer skin moist, as well. This includes sealing in your "juices" with a moisture sealing barrier.

Succulent, seductive skin holds fourteen pints of water—your good looks depend on it! These inner juices are primarily held just beneath your skin's outer layer, within the underlying dermis and the interstitial network of cells where it forms a semi-fluid gel with mucopolysaccharides and polysaccharides (sugar compounds that cosmetic companies frequently advertise). Combined with healthy collagen, it is this "juice" that makes the difference between a "grape" and a "raisin." So long as your body's water balance functions properly, the moisture in your skin's deeper layers will ensure plump, delectable skin.

The amount of water you drink can make the difference. Six to eight, full eight-ounce glasses (some authorities say 10) of mineral, spring or distilled water daily fill the quota, but check labels for low or no salt content. With sufficient water, your skin will not only plump with luscious hydration, but pore-clogging toxins and excess fluids will be washed from your body. With so many pollutants in the environment, however, it makes good sense to avoid regular tap water.

TASTY WATER RECIPES

In these days of "quicker picker uppers" and sugary fruit punches, water might need a little extra appeal. So, to add interest . . .

Try adding a **slice of lemon, lime or orange. Slices of orange and cucumber** added to water and refrigerated for an hour or two is delicious.

One or two tablespoons of raw **apple cider vinegar** added to one gallon of water tastes surprisingly good. Vinegar, preferably from your health food store, is an excellent solvent that aids digestion. Or try delicious . . .

BARLEY WATER ROYALE

Skin clarifying barley water has produced flawless complexions in Europe for centuries. Regal dining crystal overflowed with the following recipe.

½ cup pearled barley
2½ quarts boiling water
2 lemons
6 oranges (preservative and color free)
Brown sugar or honey to taste

Place the barley into a 3 quart saucepan. Over it, pour the water which has been brought to a boil. Cover and simmer on low heat for one hour. Squeeze the fruit, reserving both the juice and the skins. When cooked, strain the barley from the water. Stir in the sugar or honey. Add in the rinds from the lemons and oranges. Cool to room temperature. Remove rinds and add the juice. Refrigerate.

TO ADD MINERALS ...

... try steaming your vegetables in mineral or distilled water and drink the juice. Water from broccoli steamed with garlic and a little soy sauce makes a quick-pick-me-up broth. Artichoke, Brussels sprout and celery *waters* are great plain; also carrot-water with a little added dill. Trace Minerals Research Laboratories offer concentrated mineral drops. Two tablespoons can be added per five gallons of water.

THE MOISTURE ROBBERS

Be cautious of excessive alcoholic beverages (nutrient robbers that can age you prematurely). Take care with diuretics, laxatives, and caffeine-containing soft drinks, teas and coffee, plus medications that deplete your body of vital nutrients and cause dehydration. Watch your intake of animal fats, spices, and tannins (found in non-herbal teas and red wines)—they, too, can upset your moisture balance.

SKIN "JUICES"

Add extra moisture to your apple cheeks with fresh raw fruit and vegetable juices. They offer vitamins, minerals and other nutrients that are readily assimilable. Great for giving your digestive system a rest when fasting or ill, and incredible for reviving body, skin, and soul recovering from exhaustion, physical illness or emotional stress. *The secret is fresh. Juices must be drunk **immediately** after juicing.* Orange juice, for instance, can lose up to 50 percent of its Vitamin C within 10 minutes of juicing. Very sugary juices like pineapple should be diluted with 50 percent water, since fruit juices that are high in fructose (fruit sugar) can shock your glucose (sugar) balance. Also, as a general rule, do not combine fruits and vegetables; they require different enzymes to digest and could cause indigestion.

FRUIT JUICES

Apple. High in silicon, apple helps your skin, hair and nails. Loaded with vitamins A, B, and C, it is one of the richest sources of skin-healing potassium, and red-blood-cell-forming iron. (A bonus, Malic acid, helps dissolve and flush out cellulite).

Berries: Strawberry, Raspberry, Blueberry, Cherry. All are good sources of vitamin C and bioflavonoids, needed for cell strength and collagen production. The fresher, the better. Strawberries are high in pantothenic acid and iodine, raspberries in calcium.

Coconut. Rich in skin vitamins B and X, coconut is high in fats and carbohydrates and simple easily digested protein. Wonderful if you need to put on a few pounds or have digestive problems like stomach or duodenal ulcers or colitis. A soothing drink that is also used in cases of nerves or liver troubles.

Grape. An excellent cleanser, purifying the skin from the inside out, bioflavonoid-containing grape juice is iron rich. Adding color to an anemic complexion, grape juice helps to clear blemished skin as well. Note: Do not drink if diabetic, or if your digestive tract is inflamed.

Lemon. Historically used for clean, clear skin. High in vitamins C, B and G, also contains some A and P. Lemon is an incredible alkalizer, acid neutralizer and antiseptic, and a great sedative taken before bedtime in half an 8 ounce glass of lukewarm or tepid water. Start with half a medium lemon after dinner has been digested (at least 2 hours after eating), working up to the juice of one whole lemon. Then, brush your teeth to protect your tooth enamel. Note: If you suffer from ulcers, avoid lemon.

Melon. A good source of vitamin C and some folic acid, cantaloupe, in particular, has a very beneficial effect on eczema and other skin problems. Watermelon contains folic acid, is diuretic and cleansing. Note: Do not use melon juice in combination with other fruit juices.

Orange, Tangerine, Grapefruit. Excellent sources of vitamin C, necessary for the integrity of your skin's collagen, this citrus threesome contains a good supply of A, some B and G; also are good sources of calcium and phosphrus.

Papaya. Known for its external help in skin beautification, papaya works internally as well. High in vitamin C, papaya aids in stimulating blood flow. Enzymes, papain and papayotin help digestion.

Pineapple. An excellent body cleanser, pineapple contains the digestive-aiding enzyme bromelin. The cleaner the body, the clearer the skin.

Tomato. Classed among the citrus fruits, tomato is high in "skin" vitamin C, a good source of A and K, with some B and G. Also, a source of iodine, helpful for thyroid and glandular problems, tomato contains necessary skin minerals sodium, potassium, phosphorus, calcium, magnesium and sulphur. Also, a skin clearing blood cleanser. Hint: When eating animal-protein, tomatoes help to neutralize uric acid and help digestion; avoid tomato at a meal containing starch or sugar—an uncomfortable acid condition could result.

VEGETABLE JUICES

Aloe. A magnificent internal cleanser, drinking aloe juice adds vitality to good looks and a glowing complexion. Requiring only a few weeks to "scrub things up." a detoxifying program might include three ounces in an 8 ounce glass of water twice daily for two days, then once daily for two weeks. Continued use for general health and skin includes two ounces in an 8 ounce glass of water daily three or four times weekly. A very palatable debittered (stabilized, no need to refrigerate) aloe juice which has sugars and allantoin removed is **Aloe by George.** Aloe contains enzymes: catalase and cellulase; minerals: calcium, aluminum, iron, zinc, potassium and sodium; plus amino acids. Note: Some individuals, particularly diabetics, may develop an intolerance to aloe juice.

Beet. A powerful blood and liver cleanser, as well as a blood builder. Beet is best taken in mixes, such as carrot, or carrot and celery. Do not take more than a small wine glass at a time if taken alone or the intense cleaning action can cause nausea and dizziness. Besides helping cases of psoriasis and eczema, beet juice has been reported to help anemia, heart trouble, suppressed menstruation, poor circulation and low vitality. Prepared juice should also include the beet tops.

Cabbage. Since constipation is many times the underlying cause of skin eruptions, cabbage juice, drunk judiciously, can clear up blemishes along with the constipation. Also, a great reliever of stomach and duodenal ulcers. Not all that tasty, combining cabbage with celery or carrot and celery improves the palatability. Valuable for almost any condition of ill health, cabbage includes an abundance of almost all known minerals and is high in vitamins C, A, B and G.

Carrot. Particularly valuable for beautiful skin, hair and healthy eyes, carrot contains practically all the minerals and vitamins needed by your body, particularly beta carotene. Because of its sweet taste, it is the most popular of the vegetable juices and mixes well with any number of other vegetables. Dry skin, blemishes and dermatitis are often helped by drinking carrot juice. An excellent beverage combines carrot with celery and beet.

Celery. Another great favorite, celery's greatest value lies in its exceptionally high sodium content. If you tend to lean heavily on the refined carbohydrates (breads, pastas, cakes and cookies) and refined sugars, celery can be a lifesaver—it is a powerful dissolver of calcium deposits. Highly alkaline, it is valuable in the correction of urinary tract inflammations as well.

Cucumber. High in silicon and fluorine, essential for your skin, hair and nails. Its rich sodium content dissolves away calcium deposits, aiding in cases of high blood pressure, arthritis, hardening of the arteries, as well as gall and kidney stones.

Many types of skin eruptions have been helped by drinking **cucumber-carrot-lettuce** juice. Addition of **alfalfa** has sometimes speeded up the process. Note: When juicing, include the skins of the cucumber, but only the green portions of the lettuce—white portions are low in nutritional value.

Dandelion. Exceptionally high vitamin A, also B and G content, dandelion helps clear the complexion by cleansing the body and liver. A valuable aid to digestion, this lowly leaf balances out acid/alkaline ratio in the body and normalizes acidity. Dandelion contains almost the entire range of minerals, but is very rich in magnesium, potassium, calcium and iron. Not so lowly after all.

The incredible "grasses": Alfalfa. Iron rich alfalfa contains a balance of practically the entire range of minerals and all known vitamins. Alkaline, it produces a neutralizing effect on the intestinal tract. Wonderful for the skin, it is more palatable when mixed with carrot, or carrot and celery juice. **Barley grass.** High in calcium, iron, all the essential amino acids, vitamin C, bioflavonoids and B 12, plus minerals and enzymes. **Wheat grass.** Nutritionally rich, it is claimed to contain the greatest variety of vitamins, minerals, and trace elements of all the *greens*. Closely resembling our own red blood cells' hemoglobin, the oxygen-carrying protein contained in wheat grass is especially valuable for healthy, glowing, rosy complexions. Very sweet and potent. As with all the incredible grasses, a very little goes a long, long way. Powders for mixing can be found, or prebottled and fresh squeezed juices are available in some health food stores. See also *Anti-Aging Antioxidants*.

Green pepper. A super skin saver, green pepper is high in vitamin A, fluorine and silicon. When you juice, throw in the seeds for some extra E. Green pepper works with carrot juice to clear blemishes.

Lettuce. A good source of iron and magnesium. Among other minerals, lettuce contains silicon, sulphur and phosphorus—all essential for the proper maintenance of your skin and hair. Use only the green leaves, bleached leaves have little value. Sodium rich **Romaine** has an entirely different chemical makeup from head lettuce, but none-the-less valuable.

Parsley. Actually an herb, parsley is one of the most potent juices. Just a dash will do. Never take parsley alone and never more than an ounce at a time mixed with a high proportion of other vegetable juices, such as carrot, lettuce, spinach or celery. High in vitamin A and iron, rich in C and B, parsley also contains some E. Fabulous for improving the skin.

Potato. Juiced raw, peel and all, potato is rich in skin vitamins and minerals, particularly high in silicon, vitamins C, B, and A.

"SPRAY YOUR GRAPES" AND "OIL YOUR CUCUMBERS"

The greengrocer sprays his grapes, mists his iceberg and moistens the delicate herbs that readily dehydrate. He seals in moisture from the outside when he oils his apples and cucumbers. *Working together, oil and water keep the produce plump. So it is with your skin.*

THE OIL-WATER CONNECTION

Unlike the deeper layers, the superficial horny outer layer of your skin, the epidermis, is strongly affected by outside influences. Exposed to the sun, drying winds, changes in climate, relative humidity, seasonal fluctuations, overheated apartments, dehydrating air conditioners and pressurized airline cabins, about 3½ pints of water is given up by your outer envelope daily. Continually at risk, your skin also fights water loss instigated by airborne pollutants and many of the products that contact it. It is on this outer epidermal layer that the oil-water connection is critical. Your skin's softness and smoothness rely on it.

Without enough sebum (oil), your skin will give up too much moisture. Yet, without enough moisture, no matter how much oil is applied, your skin will not plump. Water can revive a wilted salad, but no oily dressing ever will, and lacking sufficient moisture, even very oily complexions can look blotchy and dry.

14

Like the delicate greens, your skin's outer surface is able to absorb moisture from the atmosphere. Have you noticed when splashing your face with water, getting caught in the rain, or after a bath or shower, your skin perks up, looks softer, clearer? Water is held for a while in the horny layer of cutaneous cells which look like microscopic roof tiles. Trapped between the "tiles," moisture plumps the skin which can then be sealed by your skin's own natural sebum (oils), and with the oils and moisturizers you apply.

NATURAL MOISTURIZERS

Moisture can be attracted to the skin by way of a humectant, a moisture magnet that pulls water out of the air and holds it on your skin. Mucopolysaccharides, natural skin humectants, are sugars also found in the aloe plant. Honey, a natural sugar, moisturizes as well. Alpha hydroxy acids, in fruits and milk, yogurt, buttermilk, are humectants. Water gatherers, urea and NaPCA, found naturally in the skin, can be purchased in prepared cosmetics. Unfortunately, most available cosmetics do not have sufficient amounts of these substances to make them worthwhile. NaPCA, however, can be purchased in a concentrated spray and is handy to have around (see your health food store).

Some humectants, though attracting water to the skin, will take moisture from your skin if the air is dry. Glycerin is an emollient-humectant that can cause difficulties in arid environments. However, there is one glycerin product that is excellent, particularly when you are traveling in a bone-dry airplane atmosphere, or streaking down the wind-blown ski slopes. That product is **Aqualin** and it is available in health food stores.

Collagen, billed as a rejuvenating agent in cosmetics, does plump the skin, but not as we have been led to believe. Collagen can not replace the underlying collagen structure of our skin, nor does it penetrate the outer dermis (the molecule is too large), but it is an excellent hydrator, helping to attract moisture to the skin.

CHEF'S PROTEIN COLLAGEN HYDRATOR EXTRAORDINAIRE

A unique recipe *treatment* has been suggested by the well-known cosmetic surgeon Dr. Lewis M. Feder. Bottled pre-digested protein with collagen, a once very popular "lean cuisine" dietary item, available in health food stores, can hydrate the skin for several days when used as follows: After shaking well, pour 1 or 2 tablespoons straight from the container into a small bowl. Using a clean blusher brush that you use strictly for mask applications, apply the liquid to your face, beginning at the base of your neck. Allow it to dry for one to two hours, misting lightly every 15 minutes or so with plain water or any of mixtures listed in *Moisturizing Mists* below. Rinse well with tepid water to remove. Note: This ready-made preparation can only be improved with the addition of a drop or two of your favorite essential oil or blend. See *Gourmet Ingredients*.

MOISTURIZING MISTS (Recipes)

A very practical way to maintain or replenish moisture lost throughout the day is by "misting" your face and neck. A quickie mineral water spray is marketed by Evian. And the following nutritious skin-plumping recipes can be poured into a small glass perfume atomizer for day long moisturizing.

"MIST-IFYING" TEA

Tasty, soothing and refreshing vitamin and mineral rich favorites include strong brewed herbal teas and tea blends, such as Ginseng, Rosehips (very high in vitamin C) Chamomile and Comfrey. Just brew, cool and pour into your perfume bottle.

HYDRATING HYDROSOLS

Exquisitely scented hydrosols or floral waters pamper and calm. Pour distilled water into your mister, add a drop or two of essential oil and spray away. The oils you choose can balance your sebum, rejuvenate and help reprogram your skin while supplying moisture. See *Floral Waters,* pages 122–123; and *Gourmet Ingredients* for choices.

CIDER SOAK

A sparkling combination to help maintain the integrity of your acid-mantle calls for a few drops of apple cider vinegar in mineral or distilled water. Proportions are not to exceed one teaspoon to one pint of water.

ATOMIZING ALOE

Moisturizing, healing and toning, aloe vera and mineral water is superb. Equal parts *juice* and water for **normal or combo skin.** Equal parts aloe *gel* and mineral water (or 3 parts aloe juice to 1 part water) for **acne/oily.** Equal parts aloe vera *juice and purified sea water* (available in your health food store) for **dry or mature skin.**

Your versatile "mister" can be used before applying your moisturizer, before applying makeup, afterward to set it, before exercising, oiling or creaming your face, and anytime your face needs a little lift. Always allow it to dry. Never blot.

Other natural emollient moisturizers or lubricants that seal in precious fluid and help prevent water loss, are the following user-friendly *cold pressed vegetable oils*. Here, you have a wide choice. Health food stores and some supermarkets carry the cold pressed oils.

A "SPLASH" OF OIL

At the heart of every fine salad is the right splash of oil. It should be rich and full-bodied, coating the greens while capturing the flavor of the herbs and essences in the dressing. The splash has to be fresh; the integrity of every good dressing is based on it. For our recipes, any of the following *cold pressed oils* will do wonderfully. Used alone, some of the lighter oils will do well for makeup removal, others for more intense nourishment of your skin. Just make sure the oils you use are cold pressed, which means the oils have not been extracted by a heat process that destroys the goodness. Cold pressing maintains the richness of natural vitamins, minerals and enzymes, and high essential fatty acid (vitamin F) content. Just a light coat will seal in moisture, and not to worry about pore-clogging. Cold pressed oils absorb only into the upper skin layers and, used lightly on clean skin, will not clog pores. To stay fresh, these preservative-free oils need refrigeration.

Tropical oils, such as avocado, almond, olive, peanut and coco (cocoa butter) are nondrying. Externally used, they are particularly **good for dry skin.** Containing very little linoleic and/or linolenic acids and low in iodine, they remain liquid for a long time when exposed to the air.

Semi-drying oils, particularly useful for **normal to oily skin,** include: *sesame, corn, safflower, and sunflower.* Low in linolenic acid, high in linoleic and saturated fatty acids, they dry slowly and at higher temperatures, and have a fairly high iodine number.

Drying oils for **oilier skin** include: *soy, and most nut oils.* Low in oleic acid, they dry slowly to form a film on the skin. Grown mostly in temperate climates, they have a high iodine number, are very high in unsaturated glycerides (especially linoleic and linolenic acids). *These oils are best mixed with other oils.*

Avocado oil spreads easily on the skin, contains vitamins A, B, D and E; is high in A, B1, B2, and Pantothenic acid; also a good amount of lecithin; and is absorbed fairly well. Avocado oil is very resistant to going rancid and has a light sunscreening effect. Excellent oil for dry and mature skin, as are **peach kernel** and **apricot kernel oils. Almond oil,** used in many cosmetics, creates a pleasant sensation on the skin. Relatively stable, though not as stable as avocado, it does not go rancid quickly. Used most frequently as a carrier oil in aromatherapy due to the fact that it is light, non-drying, absorbs well and is odorless.

Castor oil is a nondrying oil for dry skin, that also has laxative, cleansing effects on the skin. Rubbed into the base of the lashes, it stimulates growth.

Grapeseed oil is a carrier oil in aromatherapy massage.

Hazelnut, a rich light oil used in many facial preparations, it leaves a silky coating on the skin that feels wonderful.

Jojoba oil is actually a liquid wax. Similar to walnut oil, it spreads easily over the skin, giving it an elastic feel. Almost never going rancid, it is closest to the skin's own waxy-oil. Noncomedegenic (non-pore clogging), it is frequently used on oily-acne skins.

Olive oil has very valuable healing properties and is magic during cold weather snaps. It plumps dry skin instantly. Used traditionally in cosmetics, it is a very valuable oil. If you don't mind smelling like a salad, use it straight. And—make sure it's *extra virgin!*

Peanut oil, a good cosmetic oil, is also relatively stable. The best oil I have found is right off the top of a natural peanut butter jar. My skin just drinks it in.

Safflower oil, high in unsaturated fatty acids, especially linoleic. Inexpensive and good.

Sesame, a very nourishing oil, that is high in essential linoleic
acid. Used in many skin preparations, it has the advantage
of washing out of fabrics easily.

Shea butter, not actually an oil, it is, however, excellent for
the skin. Softening, it improves healing after injury, prevents drying and has a natural sunscreen effect. Shea butter contains allantoin, vitamin E, beta carotene and other
carotenoids. Keep Shea butter refrigerated; it spoils easily, but feels wonderful.

Soy oil is very high in linoleic acid (unsaturated fatty acid),
and contains vitamin E and lecithin.

Sunflower seed oil, low priced, contains lecithin and is very
high in linoleic acid.

Wheat germ oil, is high in vitamins E and D, contains beta
carotene and lecithin. Because it is rich in vitamin E, an
anti-scarring agent, it can be used to reduce scarring after
surgery and for facial scarring caused by very severe
acne. Wheat germ oil is a sticky oil that doesn't flow
easily. To use, add it to another oil; 25% wheat germ can
be combined with 75% almond or another light oil. A
natural anti-oxidant, wheat germ, when added to other
oils, prevents them from becoming rancid, extending their
shelf-lives by a month or two.

With the exception of wheat germ oil which is thick, any
of the above may be used singly to seal in the moisture on
your skin. High in GLA, gamma linoleic acids and linolenic
acid, capsules of evening primrose oil or black current seed
oil may also be added into lighter oils for more richness, as
well as the oil soluble vitamins A, C and E.

Cold pressed oils taken internally are equally valuable. The
essential fatty acids found in the oils cannot be made by the
body and rely on diet to supply them—that is why they are
called essential. These fatty acids reduce blood pressure, help
prevent arthritis, lower cholesterol and triglycerides, retard the

growth rate of breast cancer, aid in problems of arteriosclerosis, are needed in the treatment of coronary heart disease, are essential for the normal growth and development of the brain, and are useful in the treatment of eczema and psoriasis, and more. Internally, the most essential of the fatty acids is linoleic, requiring 10% to 20% of your total daily calorie intake. See *Essential Fatty Acids*.

With sufficient surface hydration and internal moisture, you will be able to seal in your "juices" with replenishing oils, while feeding and protecting your skin's protective acid mantle. So, spray your delicate greens and hydrate your goodies, but before you oil your cucumbers and seal in those "juices," make sure your skin is nibbling clean.

"NIBBLING" CLEAN!

Irresistibly edible skin is clean, clean, clean! No roquefort, herbal or vinegarette can penetrate grit in the parsley or gunk on the green peppers, and no intensive blemish-clearing wrinkle-erasing "recipe" can be absorbed through clogged, constipated skin. Only nibbling clean skin can absorb your nutritious formulations. And to be munchable, skin must be clean not only from **the outside in,** but from **the inside out** as well.

The body's largest organ of elimination, your skin flushes out wastes and toxins through its pores. When you build up more "grunge" than your skin, kidneys and liver (also cleansing and filtering organs) can handle, lumps and bumps, welts, blemishes and pimples result.

Toxin and sludge makers include those infamous refined sugars and refined carbohydrates, fried foods, indigestible animal fats, alcohol and caffeine. Go easy on the french fries and potato chips, milled grains and flour, full fatted ice creams, cookies, cakes and candies. Red flag chocolate, colas, coffee and other caffeine containers. *Over a period of time, improper diet, particularly one lacking in protein (sometimes the result of fad dieting), and deficient in vitamins A, C and E, zinc and silicon leads to collagen breakdown, and premature sagging and wrinkling.*

Your skin directly reflects your entire physical condition. Nibbling clean means nibbling on the right foods. A magnetic glowing complexion is the direct result of a clean, sludge-free and healthy inner you. Munch on those vitamin and mineral rich fresh fruits and veggies. Be sure to balance in sufficient protein—*your skin's collagen and elastin are proteins, and all your body's enzymes are protein. Without enough protein, your body will begin to deplete the protein in your skin and muscle. Don't forget whole grains and complex carbohydrates.* Many over-oily, over-dry or problematic conditions clear rapidly with a change in diet.

Fill your bowl with only first rate ingredients, including fresh whole ripe fruits and veggies, nuts, whole grains, herbs and legumes. Be sure to include your 6 to 8, eight ounce glasses of water a day along with your fresh raw fruit and vegetable juices along with whichever proteins work best for you. See *Plant Food Plus: Feeding Your Skin From Within.*

SCRUB THOSE CARROTS, PEEL THOSE POTATOES!

Cleansing the outside can be as simple as a teaspoon full of cold pressed salad oil.

*For a **light morning freshening** on a makeup free face . . . place a teaspoon or more of vegetable oil in the palm of your hand—you will find that you select your oils according to the weather, the climate and the condition or type of your skin. Carefully rub your hands together to distribute the oil evenly on both palms. Beginning at the base of your neck, spread the oil onto your skin using gentle upward and outward strokes. Work up and over your cheeks, circle around your eyes, moving from the outside corner of your eyes to the inside on the under eye, and on the upper eye work from the inner corners out. Cover your entire face with a thin oily film. This dissolves the oily dirt. Now, with a dampened cosmetic pad or clean (never reuse without washing) facial cloth, gently remove the oil and grit with the same motions used to apply the oil. Use as many dampened pads as needed.*

When finished, splash your face with warm water to open your pores, about 20 splashes should do it.

Note: Use only vegetable oils. Avoid mineral, baby oil, or vaseline containing products no matter how well they are advertised. Read labels. Petroleum production leftovers can clog pores and cause a rebound effect. Actually robbing your skin of nutrients, after a time, they will dry the very skin they are thought to be protecting.

For a little cell sloughing stimulation, you may wish to add . . . *a heaping tablespoon or two of plain oatmeal dampened with water, plus a little witch hazel and water if your skin tends to the oily side. Work upward and outward, as in the application of your oil, adding little circular movements. Linger over the oilier areas of your face, particularly the nose area where blackheads may be lurking. The oatmeal acts to blot up excess oil and is a mild exfoliant that removes dead skin cells. When finished, splash with lots more warm water.*

Cleansing in this way removes the two types of surface dirt, water soluble and oil soluble. The grit on the parsley can be rinsed off with water, but the gunk on the peppers needs another approach. And, who would believe the barest bones skin cleansing ingredients can simply include a handful of oatmeal and a little vegetable oil? These ingredients can be used by almost all complexions.

For makeup removal . . . *Saturate two cosmetic puffs in water. Squeeze out the excess. Then, drip a few drops of vegetable oil onto the pads. Use them to carefully and gently remove your eye makeup, stroking over your closed lids, one eye at a time. Stroke downward toward the lashes and do not rub. The delicate skin and capillaries in this area can be easily damaged. The oil will dissolve the makeup and the pad will remove it.*

When your upper eye area is completed, moisten and oil as many pads as necessary to clear the makeup from the rest of your face, always working in upward and outward motions. Remember, also, to work from the outside corner of your eye to the inside corner when touching the under eye areas. After removing all dirt and makeup, splash your face with cold water.

At this time you may want to incorporate a relaxing, muscle toning, rejuvenating aromatic face massage. See *The Wilted Salad Supreme,* or incorporate the total rebalancing healing luxury of the **Facelift Naturally** finger pressure face lift.

Cleansing at the end of the day involves makeup removal and for most skins a little deeper cleansing is in order. Night is when your skin regenerates more rapidly. So, you will want it spanking clean and ready to absorb your marinades and dressings.

Now is also a perfect time to deep clean with a cell sloughing preparation. Also known as deep pore cleansers and exfoliants, skin renewal formulations serve to remove pore clogging dry dead skin cells from the outermost surface of your skin, the stratum corneum.

Natural, at-home exfoliant preparations are one of two types: *grainy* mechanical cleansers such as oatmeal, or acid-enzyme peels. The grainy cleansers literally *sand* off the upper dry dead cells, fine lines, and all. The acids or enzymes *dissolve* the "glue" that holds the cells together, allowing the dry old dead cells to be rinsed away. Both stave off wrinkles and blemishes by allowing your cells to regenerate more quickly, stimulating circulation and oxygen in your skin, as they unclog pores and allow the free flow of skin oils. Continued use of exfoliants can encourage your skin to renew itself at a faster rate. Whichever approach you choose, exfoliation is always undertaken on a clean face.

MECHANICAL EXFOLIANTS

The following recipes are mild formulations that can be used daily, however very oily skin or acne-oily, should limit abrasive scrubs to three times a week. Although effective deep pore cleansers, they also stimulate oil production. Extremely dry or sensitive skin may prefer a non-abrasive Acid-Enzyme Peel, listed under **Fruity Peels,** and very sensitive skin with broken capillaries will avoid abrasive peels altogether.

YOGURT-MEAL SCRUB

1 teaspoon oatmeal
1 teaspoon honey
1 teaspoon corn meal
1 teaspoon yogurt
½ teaspoon vegetable oil (optional for dry skin)

Mix all ingredients together and apply to a freshly cleaned face. If your skin is sensitive or extra dry, you may wish to apply a thin layer of vegetable oil before starting. Extremely sensitive skins should avoid scrubs altogether.

To begin, evenly distribute about 2 tablespoons of the mixture in the palms of your hands and apply in an upward, outward and circular motion, starting at the base of your neck. You will feel a light tingling sensation as your fingertips gently move the abrasive mixture over your skin. Working in this way gets under the horny epidermal cells, which are arranged like overlapping roof tiles or shingles. They are loosened, removed and easily washed away. Massage very gently for a good minute. Let your recipe do the work, taking care not to press your scrub into your skin. Pressure could easily break capillaries and damage the new emerging cells. Rinse with warm water splashing your face at least 20 to 30 splashes.

Hint: Wheatena, very finely ground almond meal, or jojoba beans may be used in place of the cornmeal. For more exotic fare, powdered alfalfa, ginseng, comfrey, spirulina, kelp, or any number of powdered roots and herbs may also be added. Avoid nut or seed shells, such as apricot or walnut, these can scratch your delicate skin.

VANISHING GRANULES

Deep pore scrubs can incorporate **fine grained mineral rich sea salt and/or** slightly antibacterial **sugar granules** that dissolve as you ''scrub,'' protecting your skin from abrasion. Very effective when used alone, they, too, may be substituted for or added to the corn meal in the above recipe.

MASQUE ALMANDINE

A super home peel, particularly effective for oily skin.

1 tablespoon finely ground almonds
1 tablespoon unfiltered honey
1 egg white

Combine the almonds, honey and egg white.

To apply: Starting at the base of the neck, coat your skin with the mixture as you would with any mask. Do not scrub. Allow to dry for 15–20 minutes. To remove: First, dampen with warm water. Then, apply enough water to massage for 1 minute in upward, outward, circular motions. Avoid the eye area. Rinse very well.

Note: Avoid commercial exfoliating masks that need to be rubbed off. Besides leaving a wax or paraffin base that requires additional cleansing, the rubbing can irritate most skins. Both are particularly detrimental to sensitive or acneic skin.

OATMEAL SCANDINAVIANNE

Expanding on the basics, Ole Hendricksen, one of Hollywood's top skin care specialists, suggests little soap-like sachets.

12 heaping tablespoons oatmeal
⅓ cup witch hazel
2 heaping tablespoons plain yogurt

Using your blender, shred the oatmeal for a few seconds. Stop the blender. Shake to redistribute the oats, then shred again for another few seconds. Place the oats into a mixing bowl, adding the remaining ingredients. Mix well. Cut 6 pieces of cheesecloth, 7 × 8 inches each.

To make the sachets: Layer three pieces of the cloth, making two piles. Divide the mixture in half, placing each half on each of the two layered piles. Tie a string around each sachet taking care not to squeeze out the contents. Place in a tight container and refrigerate. Each will remain fresh for three consecutive days.

Before using: Add a little warm water to soften refrigerated sachets.

When finished, splash your face again with cold water. Apply an astringent or toner depending on your skin type, and a moisturizing *dressing* if needed.

Hint: The oatmeal can be moistened with almost any drinkable liquid from buttermilk to apple or aloe juice with nutritional advantage. A little moisturizing vegetable oil or mayonnaise can be added if needed for very dry or sensitive skin.

THE STICKY MASK

An entertaining exfoliation method that also moisturizes includes ...

1 tablespoon of raw unfiltered honey

When shopping for unfiltered honey, avoid labels that read "unheated." It is not the same as "unfiltered" and may, in fact, be actually heated below a specified temperature. Raw unfiltered honey is cloudy in appearance—what you are seeing is all the natural active enzymes and important nutrients that heating and filtering eliminate. *For a little extra rejuvenation try sage honey mixed with a little powdered alfalfa and powdered ginseng that can be found in capsules in your health food store.*

To apply: Dab the honey over your throat and face. Then begin to gently tap. Continue tapping for a minute or two. As you tap, the circulation in your face increases with the gentle massage and the dry dead surface cells are lifted off with the sticky honey. Rinse thoroughly.

FRUITY PEELS

Having received the lion's share of PR lately, no one "cookin'" in skin care has missed the alpha hydroxy titillation sweeping the cosmetic industry. The AHAs (alpha hydroxy acids) actually encompass a broad range of organic acids including the also familiar sugarcane derived glycolic acid.

Actually known for centuries, Cleopatra's famed skin was the result of the alpha hydroxy acid—*lactic acid found in the sour milk* she used in her baths. Ladies in the French Court swore by anti-wrinkle agent *tartaric acid,* daubing their smooth, glowing complexions with clarifying *old wine.*

In fact, if you have an **orange** (*citric acid*), **lemon, grape,**

grapefruit, or an **apple** in the house, a can of **tomatoes,** a carton of **yogurt, fermented buttermilk,** or wine that has *turned,* you have the makings of an AHA peel.

Equally effective are the enzyme based exfoliants that include the powerfully clarifying **papaya** (*papain enzyme*) and **pineapple** (*bromelin enzyme*).

To begin "peeling": *simply apply the pulp or juice of any one or more of the preceding fruits and/or beverages directly to your face for fifteen to twenty minutes.*

Hints: *Canned tomatoes are more acidic than fresh and, green papaya is more active than the ripe fruit. The inner skin of the papaya can be used along with the fruit to exfoliate, combining the mechanical abrading action with the enzymatic. Although not an acid or enzyme peel, the inner skin of an oil-rich avocado is a terrific mechanical exfoliant, sanding and smoothing, while adding vitamin E.* **Always rinse thoroughly.**

While *mashed fruit, juices and beverages can be used alone, you may prefer to mix your fruity peel with a little clay for substance. Depending on the amount of clay used, drier skins may enjoy the addition of a little vegetable oil and/or honey in the mixture.*

Natural, gentle, at-home fruity peels work their culinary magic very slowly. They not only encourage new cell growth, they lighten sun or age spots, fade scars, eliminate fine lines and wrinkles, balance out dryness, uneven pigmentation, and acne, as well as unclog pores. You will not actually see your skin redden, crust or peel as in a sun burn or a deep skin peel that is given by a physician using high concentrations of chemical acids. There is no recuperation time, nor is there the danger of uneven pigmentation, burning, compromising the immune system (your skin is your first line of defense), over-thinning aging skin or other tenuous results. Either **enzyme or acid based,** the gentle at-home fruity peels are meant to be used daily.

Before applying any fruit or vegetable preparation to your skin always test a small area first. While you may be able to eat certain foods, some may cause a reaction when applied to your skin.

WILTED SALAD SUPREME

FACIAL FOR ONE OR TWO

Sheer luxury, the *Wilted Salad Supreme* can be as elaborate or as simple as you desire. A feast for the skin and a feast for the soul, with a little candlelight, soft music and the exquisite aroma of essential oils, a cleansing, toning, rejuvenating ritual for one can be an exciting and relaxing experience for two.

The Wilted Salad Supreme has six basic steps.

1. *Initial cleansing.*
2. *The aromatherapy, or gentle oil massage.*
3. *The facial sauna, compress, or aromatic mist.*
4. *Deep pore scrub, or acid-enzyme exfoliation, or facial mask.*
5. *Toning.*
6. *Moisturizing.*

The herbs, marinades and dressings that you apply in each step will depend on what will balance your skin type, balance the activity of your oil glands, nourish, moisturize, dry, tighten, and remineralize. The basic facial can be done once or twice a week.

STEP BY STEP

1. **Cleansing or washing.** Cleanse as usual. Do not apply makeup. *If you are omitting The Light Facial Massage*

(Step 2), and are not using a facial scrub or a face mask, apply your "Fruity Peel" now, and go to Step 3.
2. **Light Facial Massage.** A plain cold pressed vegetable oil will do—*a scented aroma massage does it better!*

SWEET SCENTED SEDUCTION:
The Aroma Massage

Strictly for you, my pampered chef—massaging with essential oils is pure luxury. For special blends, see *Exotic Marinades*.

Setting the Stage. Easy listening music and candlelight enhance the relaxation of this delicate light massage.

Starting. To begin, lift the hair away from your, or your partner's, face and neck. If massaging a partner, he or she should be lying down, completely relaxed with head, neck and shoulders free of clothing. Pour about ½ teaspoon of scented oil into the palm of your hand. If this doesn't adequately cover the face and the neck, use a little more, some skins just drink in the oil.

Stroking. Run through the movements several times in your mind or over your own face, especially if you are undertaking a massage for two. You will want to know your way around, because the second your hands touch the skin, your movements must be continuous and fluid.

With both hands under the chin, fingers relaxed, fingertips touching, wrists supple, hands pliable, stroke out and upward to the ears. Return to center. Now, using your entire hands, glide across the face toward the temples. Then, move gently under the eyes, up the bridge of the nose, over the eyebrows, gently under the eyes again, and once more up the bridge of the nose, over the forehead to the hairline. Palm over the forehead, and over the eyebrows to the hairline several more times.

Then, in one continuous stroke, move down the nose, chin and throat, oiling the neck as you stroke. Without pause, return to your starting point, repeating the same movements as before, only this time use only one finger of each hand to circle the eyes. Be sure your movements are light, fluid and flowing. Complete the stroke several more times and return to the neck. Now, using your whole hand in slow, gentle, rhythmic strokes, go over the face and neck several times, your movements becoming lighter and lighter. Finish with a light palming of the forehead and light finger vibration over the eyes. Heaven, yes?

The natural warmth stimulated by the massage opens the pores and aids the penetration of the essential oils. Leave the oils on the skin about 15 minutes to allow for full penetration. During this time, warm compresses of mineral water, or distilled water that contains *essential oils, or hydrosols* (calming floral waters left over from the distillation of essential oils) should be applied to the face, or facial steaming undertaken. See *Essential Oils—Resources* in the back of the book for distributors of essential oils.

3. **Steaming the Face *or* the Penetrating Compress.** Based on the principle that intense sweating will loosen debris in the pores, flush out body toxins, and accelerate cell regeneration while hydrating the skin, steaming the face works incredibly well for everyone **but** *the following skin types: very sensitive, those with Acne Rosacea or anyone with broken capillaries (the steam dilates capillaries). If your skin is sensitive, prone to acne rosacea or has even one broken capillary, use a warm penetrating compress instead.*

THE PENETRATING COMPRESS

Cut your compress from a piece of white flannel or toweling, leaving holes for the eyes and under the nose. Saturate the compress in a bowl of comfortably warm mineral water, or water to which essential oils have been added, 2 to 4 drops of essential oil depending on your skin type. See *Gourmet Ingredients;* or herbs as below. Saturate the compress by dipping it close to the surface of the water so that much of the floating oil is absorbed into the compress. Squeeze out the excess water.

Your eyes should always be slightly cooler than your face, so a slice of Cucumber could be placed over each eye—or cool moist tea bags of Chamomile or Rosehips, or cotton pads dipped in Rosewater or Lavender water. Relax and let the oils and herbs penetrate for about 15 to 20 minutes.

STIMULATING STEAM

More extractive than a compress, this method is particularly effective for oily, acneic or congested complexions. If using the steam method, begin to prepare this section of your facial as you remove your makeup, so it will be ready directly after cleansing or massage. Herbal steams can include loose or herbal teas in bags, or essential oils.

THE HERBAL STEAM

Option 1. Place in the bottom of a large 2½ or 3 quart bowl, either 2 bags or two tablespoons each of the following teas: Ginseng (if you prefer, 1 capsule of ground ginseng root), Chamomile, Comfrey, and Rosehips; or mix and match with Lavender, Sage, Rosemary and/or Peppermint. Now place the bowl where it is comfortably accessible, on the kitchen table or bathroom counter.

Option 2. Swiss Kriss, a ready combination of 15 herbs in a cleansing detoxifying laxative tea may be used. In health foods, it is available loose or in tablets (use 1 tablet or 1 or 2 tablespoons of loose herbs). Place the herbs you select in the bowl, and fill it with near boiling water. Or try . . .

THE AROMATIC MIST

If using essential oils in lieu of dried herbs or teas, allow the water to cool slightly before adding 3 to 5 drops of one, or a blend of all, or several of the following: Chamomile, Lavender, Rosemary, Peppermint. The oils are highly volatile and will evaporate very quickly in the heated water. See *Gourmet Ingredients*.

Sit about 12" or so from the bowl, or facial sauna, with a towel draped over your head to capture the steam for about 10 to 15 minutes or for as long as the steam lasts. Take care not to burn yourself with the steam. The hot steamy vapors will clear sinuses, feel wonderful, smell wonderful and be wonderful for your skin.

As your lean over the bowl or your sauna, allow your head to hang down, totally releasing the cares of the day, and the stress in the spinal disks of your neck as well. When the mist has cleared, you may want to use a deep pore cleanser, or continue on to the mask. Or, if you have used a *Fruity Peel,* now is the time to rinse it off.

4. **Undressing the Skin.** Undressing the skin can be done in one of three ways.
   A. Deep pore cleansing.
   B. Acid-enzyme exfoliation or Fruity Peel.
   C. Face mask or pack.

If you have already applied a *Fruity Peel,* go to Step 5. If not, continue with either *Deep pore cleansing* or apply a *Face mask.*

DEEP PORE CLEANSING

A *grainy scrub* is best undertaken while your pores are open. It should follow immediately after steaming. An easy scrub for all skin types combines equal parts yogurt, oatmeal, honey and cornmeal. For other options, see *Scrub Those Carrots, Peel Those Potatoes*.

THE FACE MASK

The face mask serves to deep clean, feed, and also calm the skin by tightening and closing the pores. Basic ingredients for a face mask recipe can include: plain yogurt (cleansing, toning, extractive, yet mild enough for all complexions), clay and/or oatmeal (both extractive, and nourishing), brewer's yeast (optional), fruits, vegetables, vegetable oil (depending on skin type), and herbs or essential oils, vitamins can also be added, particularly A and E. If it's healthy and edible, it's wearable. See *Masques de Maison* and *Masques Exotique*. Whatever your selection, apply your mask for 20 minutes, then rinse off thoroughly with tepid water.

5. **Toning.** To complete your facial, mist, splash or pat a toner on your face to further encourage pore tightening. See *Moisturizing Mists* and/or *Resurrection Dressings*.
6. **Moisturizing.** After toning, moisturize with a *Day Dressing,* or a *Night Soak* or an intensive care *Monday Marinade*. If applying makeup, wait for at least 20 minutes to apply.

II.
"WHAT'S IN
THE BOWL?":
YOUR SKIN TYPE

THE PERFECT DRESSING

The perfect dressing is the sauce that suits your skin today. Tomorrow, your lip-smakin' tasty recipe may well need a splash of this or a dash of that to balance temporary changes in diet, seasons and hormones. Oily moisture-laden summer skins bathe in a light sauce, while the demands of winter require hardier fare. And an overindulgence in fried foods, sugar, caffeine, or alcohol can present challenges to the most masterful chef's marinade.

Throughout the weeks, months, and years, oil, moisture, hormonal cycles and nutritional needs fluxuate. In time, overactive teenage skin will wind down, craving more lubrication and moisture, and perhaps, herbal hormone support, as well. No one food supplies every nutritional requirement, and the dressing that works like a charm today, may need some major revamping tomorrow. Isn't it wonderful to have a refrigerator and pantry filled with choices?

Elaborate or simple, the "dressings" you choose for your salad always depend on the ingredients in the bowl. So, let's get down to it. What's in the bowl? What is your skin type today? *Regular Tossed Normal? Crouton Dry? Olive Oily? Chef's T-Zone Combo? OverRipe Fruit? Marinading Mature? FridgeWorn Devitalized? PotLuck Acne? Or, OverSeasoned Sensitive?* Even if you think you know your skin type, read through each description. You may have some surprises.

TYPING YOUR SKIN

*Skin is typed by **oil content**: all over normal, normal-dry, dry, normal-oily, oily, oily-acneic, or combination—some parts dry and some parts oily; by **water content**—normal, dehydrated or over-hydrated; by **vitality**—normal, devitalized, or overactive; by age and ability to regenerate—mature; and by **sensitivity**— any skin type can be sensitive, inflamed or irritated all of the time or some of the time.*

Many complexions are cross-types—maybe that's why they are called *complex*-ions. **Marinading Mature** may have a great deal in common with **Crouton Dry** or **OverSeasoned Sensitive** and sometimes **PotLuck Acne.** A **Regular Tossed Normal** may, in fact, be a **Chef's T-Zone Combo.** And, at times, we can all be **Fridge Worn Devitalized.** Throughout a lifetime, it is possible to experience, many, if not all of these variations at one time or another, and some in combination.

With all skin types, the same simple principles apply. Whether you are **Crouton Dry,** or **PotLuck Acne,** your basics are not all that different from a **Regular Tossed Normal. OverSeasoned Sensitive** and problem skins must be extra cautious. In some cases, important variations do exist in the balancing formulations and care in which you select your nutritional sauces, tonics, marinades, dressings and masks.

So, before we start really mixin', let's find out—
What is in that bowl?!

MEASURING THE OIL

If you are in doubt about your skin's oil balance. The following should help.

1. **Wash** *your face with lukewarm water and a mild soap. Dove is easy to obtain and will do nicely. Soap-free* **Lowila** *(Westwood Pharmaceutical) and* **Aveenobar** *(Cooper Laboratory), are also good selections.*
2. **Rinse well** *with comfortably hot water.*
3. **Pat dry.**
4. **Leave your face "undressed"** *for two or three hours.*
5. **Cut onion skin or facial blotting paper** *into 4 one-inch squares. Mark one "forehead," another "cheek," "nose" and "chin."*
6. **Blot.** *Place each one on the appropriate area for a slow count of ten, enough time to register the oil content.*
7. **Examine** *the papers in good light.*

If no oil appears on the paper, that area is *dry*. If the trace of oil is faint, the area is *normal*. If the paper is marked with more than a faint trace of oil, that area is *oily*. And heavy oil marks indicate a *very oily* skin.

Still in doubt? Remain dressing free for several more hours and repeat the test. Then without washing, test again in the morning. This will give you a pretty good gauge of your oil flow.

Regular Tossed Normal. You are basically balanced overall; no areas are excessively oily. There may be some light oil in the T-zone—*forehead, nose and chin* at the end of the day and while exercising or perspiring, but the area is never overoily.

Crouton Dry. Your skin is inadequate in oil production and, most probably, dehydrated as well. Papers will be oil free and your skin will look dull and chalky. If gently scraped with a fingernail, dry cells will probably flake off.

Chef's T-Zone Combo. You will show oil in the T-Zone—*forehead, nose,* and sometimes the paper marked *chin,* are stained with oil.

Olive Oily. No guessing here, your skin will stain all papers consistently and obviously with oil.

REGULAR TOSSED NORMAL

Are you a **Regular Tossed Normal**? Your skin appears moist and smooth. Without looking shiny-oily, enough sebum is produced to prevent dehydration, but not so much that pores clog. Regular Tossed Normal looks neither porcelain-fine, nor coarse or thick. Pores are visible, but not large, and never, or almost never, clogged. In general, Regular Tossed Normal is blemish free and no teenage acne scars are visible. Not perfect, but as close as you can get. If you have mildly oily skin as a teenager, you will, most likely, have normal adult skin.

If, however, you over-burden normal skin with heavy creams and oils, you will, of course, ''sprout'' pimples. Over-washing for a time or exposure to drying products such as, harsh detergents, alcohol astringents, or a drying environment, will dry, chap and irritate your skin. But, as soon as the situation is corrected, your skin will soon return to normal.

If your are a Regular Tossed Normal, Congratulations! You have the kitchen all to yourself. Every scrumptious recipe in this cookbook is yours for the trying.

Read also *Chef's T-Zone Combo,* just in case you might be a mild combination skin. Combination complexions sometimes believe their skins are normal, so sufficient caution isn't taken to control oil in the T-Zone.

CROUTON DRY

Crouton Dry, you are most likely translucent, very fine, close-grained and beautiful when young. Porcelain-like in appearance, your pores are barely visible. Take extra care, however, dry skin tends to deteriorate more readily than any other if not lovingly tended. Fine lines will appear around the mouth and eyes early in life.

If you are Crouton Dry, the sebaceous glands lying just beneath the surface of your skin do not produce sufficient lubrication, so protection from environmental fluctuations and pollutants is lacking. Usually noticed in the early twenties, when oil production begins to slow, the tendency toward "dry" can be seen first on the arms and lower legs, areas that have fewer sebaceous glands.

Or your dry skin can come and go, depending on the environment. The skin's outermost layer, the stratum corneum, normally contains 10% to 20% water. When the water saturation drops below 10%, cells parch and become brittle. Moist summer humidity or dry winter wind can make a decided difference.

Often very delicate, blemished Crouton Dry complexions are the result of sensitivity. But not to fear, dry skin can be kept moisturized. Wrinkles can be easily removed or avoided, and your fine little pores are well worth the extra care.

FALSE DRY SKIN

If your Crouton Dry skin does not fit the descriptions, dehydration may be brought on by the care your face is receiving. The products you are applying may be the cause. "False" dry skin can be cosmetically induced with the application of heavy pore-clogging creams, resulting in underfunctioning, sluggish oil glands and constipated skin. Overscrubbing, applications of alcohol or skin-drying masks and detergents can also cause skin to dehydrate.

What does or does not go into your body must also be considered. Inadequate water intake or heavy alcohol consumption will dehydrate the skin. After an occasional night on the town, be sure to drink sufficient fluids to replace those lost and lightly steam your skin to allow for surface moisture absorption.

Excessive use of caffeine, found in coffee, chocolate, tea, cocoa and cola drinks, dehydrates. Don't squeeze into those jeans too often with the help of diuretics. Laxatives, used in excess, may cause dehydrating diarrhea, and prolonged use can cause a chemical blood imbalance. Many prescription drugs dehydrate. Be sure to ask your doctor for the side effects of any drug you are taking. When your body dehydrates, your electrolytes are upset, important minerals, such as calcium and potassium are lost, as well as trace minerals and vitamins. Take care with what you eat and drink.

AGING DRY SKIN

With age, all skin becomes drier—hormonal changes contribute to oil production slowdown. With time, skin also thins, diminishing its water-holding ability. As the years progress, the natural mucopolysaccharides that help hold moisture on your skin decline. Other negative contributions can be made by ultraviolet radiation and overexposure to the sun. At a moisture disadvantage from the start, thin Crouton Dry must be carefully tended, especially in the sunlight. See also *Marinading Mature*.

DIETARY HELP

Drink plenty of water. Make sure you are getting your full 6 to 8, 8-ounce glasses of water a day. Add unsaturated fatty acids to your diet in the form of cold pressed vegetable oils. Start with two tablespoons a day. This can be part of your salad dressing. Linseed oil may also be purchased in capsule form.

Some people have difficulty assimilating oils. You may want to try a tablespoon of olive oil with half a grapefruit first thing in the morning, then wait a half hour before eating. It may not sound too inviting, but it is an excellent gall bladder flush that has helped several friends avoid gall bladder surgery and add oils to their skin, as well. This can be eaten on a regular basis as long as necessary.

Vitamin A deficiency. Dry skin can often be the first sign of vitamin A deficiency. If you have "gooseflesh" on your arms and legs, particularly the inner thighs that doesn't go away, check your diet. Foods high in vitamin A include: yellow veggies, fish, liver, milk, margarine.

Ye olde tyme **cod liver oil,** high in vitamin A, is a total body lubricant from your blood vessels to your brain. If you are game, you may really reap results, many a dry skin has. The following is to be taken on an empty stomach first thing in the morning or just before bedtime.

Mix **1 tablespoon cod liver oil** *(flavored is available, mint, cherry. . . .)* with **2 tablespoons of whole milk** *for best results—if milk is a problem, fresh-squeezed orange juice is second best. Shake well in a small container to emulsify the oil* *with the milk. Note: Taking cod liver oil capsules will not do the same thing.*

Vitamin B deficiency. Cracked skin around the lips may indicate a B deficiency. Bs are found in yeast, liver and whole grains.

Make sure your diet also includes plenty of **vitamin E** foods: leafy greens, whole grains, liver, cold pressed vegetable oils. **Sulfur,** found in eggs, garlic, onions, asparagus and the amino acid **L-cysteine** (can be found in pill form), keeps the skin smooth and dewy. The herb **chaparral** heals and softens the skin. It is available in pills or tea.

See also *Plant Food Plus, Anti-Aging Anti-Oxidants* and *Skin Juices.*

SPECIAL CARE

When cleansing, take care not to strip your skin of natural oils with harsh routines. The oatmeal and oil wash can work very well for most dry skin. Avoid heavy grainy scrubs. For morning cleansing, you may opt only for a mild oil cleansing with extra virgin olive oil. The naturally occurring squalene in **olive oil** is fabulous for dry skin. Be sure the water you use is never hot. And, always remember, less is more in skin care. This applies emphatically for dry and sensitive skin.

Astringent-toners containing alcohol, witch hazel or citrus extracts as the primary ingredients are *no-nos.* A **light toner,** such as cucumber juice or aloe and seawater, is fine. Always use a **moisturizer;** avoid harsh drying wind and wear **sun screen** *SPF 15.* For overheated rooms in winter, a **pan of hot water** on the radiator or a **humidifier** will balance the moisture. Air conditioning systems can be equally drying, as can frequent saunas. Mist your skin often during the day. See *Moisturizing Mists.* Dehydrating beverages, demineralizing laxatives and diuretics should be avoided. See also *The Moisture Robbers.*

Applied topically, **aloe vera** is very healing. Collagen is an excellent hydrator. See *Chef's Collagen Protein Hydrator Extraordinaire*. *Lanolin* has helped many a dry complexion, but many other skins are sensitive to this product. Your own skin will dictate your best approach. See also *Monday Marinades* for intensive care formulas. If you are over 35, see *Marinading Mature*.

RECIPES

CARESSING COMPOTE

Masks of mashed banana, cooked carrot, melon (especially cantaloupe), and avocado are particularly comforting for Crouton Dry complexions.

Any one or two applied directly to the skin with the addition of a little optional wheat germ oil and/or honey, left on for about 20 minutes is gluttonous luxury.

ALOE ADE

2 ounces of aloe in 8-oz glass of water drunk daily, until dryness is improved. Then, three times weekly. See also Skin Juices.

APPLE WHIP

1 medium size apple
½ teaspoon whipping cream
1 tablespoon honey

Core, pare, chop and mash the apple. Add cream and honey. Apply to a clean face for 20 minutes. Rinse thoroughly with warm water, then with cold. Apply toner.

HONEY HYDRATOR

1 egg yolk
1 tablespoon honey
1 tablespoon cold pressed vegetable oil
5 drops apple cider vinegar

Mix the egg yolk, honey, oil and vinegar together. Apply to a clean face for 20 minutes. Rinse thoroughly with warm water, then cold. Apply toner.

HONEY-MAYO MARINADE

1 egg yolk
1 teaspoon honey
1 teaspoon mayonnaise
1 tablespoon buttermilk

Mix yolk, honey, mayo and buttermilk together and apply to a clean face for 20 minutes. Rinse thoroughly with warm water, then cold. Apply toner.

See also *Dressings for All Occasions*.

OVERSEASONED SENSITIVE

OverSeasoned Sensitive? Any complexion can fall victim, not only the traditional image of the porcelain-thin fair skin that usually comes to mind. If your skin is sensitive, I hope you were born a detective. OverSeasoned Sensitive complexions must be on guard; many factors can be irritants. What works for you one day may irritate the next. Some days your skin will react badly to practically everything that touches it causing itching, burning, stinging, chafing and other discomforts.

Weather changes or environmental factors, many times, can precipitate an incident and instigate a chain reaction resulting in contact dermatitis. Consider, as an example, three factors: cold outside air, a hot bath and a particular perfume. Without the cold air and hot bath, the particular perfume poses no problem, but with the other factors, i.e., cold air plus hot bath, the skin becomes sensitive to the perfume. Sometimes the chain has more links than a super sleuth can detect.

Many sensitive skins react most unfavorably to winter's cold dry air, wind and dehydrating central heating or cooling systems. In fact, some of the most common skin irritants are environmental.

Nonenvironmental skin sensitizers or allergens are other factors to consider, as are foods and emotions.

CONTACT-SENSITIVE SKIN

Allergic? Easily sensitized by contact? Irritating fabrics should be avoided and harsh residues left by detergents eliminated. Wash clothes in low sudsing soaps like Ivory.

If you easily sensitize to products applied to your skin, it is important to test and retest, since you can build up a tolerance to a product, sometimes after months of trouble-free use. Before using any new preparation, including the recipes in this book, patch-test on your forearm undisturbed for 24 hours. If redness or swelling results, avoid the preparation. If contemplating a store-bought perfume or cosmetic, try to test it in the store before buying the product. Be particularly cautious with fragrances, the most common allergen in skin care products. Avoid coal tars, especially found in toners. Lanolin is on the allergen list, and preservatives can also be irritating, as well as detergents in facial cleansers; most often seen are sodium laurel sulfate and laureth 4.

Among the ingredients the FDA classes as safe are: allantoin, calamine, cocoa butter, glycerine, kaolin, shark liver oil (contains squalene, also found in olive oil) and zinc oxide.

For perfumes, you might consider using diluted essential oils which incur almost no sensitivity problems, although citrus oils and occasionally eucalyptus can be irritating. Avoid clove and cinnamon unless highly diluted; they are known skin irritants.

See *Exotic Marinades.*

Your best bet: Read labels and always test a new product on a small area before applying. Even if you can eat it, sometimes you can't wear it—the reverse is also true.

FOOD SENSITIVE SKIN

Diet can play a major role in sensitive skin. Blemishes or irritable skin can result from negative food reactions. *Some foods that are likely to cause sensitivities include dairy products (quiche, whole egg mayo, cakes and cookies made with egg and/or milk), wheat products, shellfish and seafood, chocolate, cola nuts (soft drink flavoring), peanuts and soy, strawberries, oranges and tomatoes, processed and refined foods.* Reactions can include hives to eczema to puffy eyes.

EMOTIONALLY SENSITIVE SKIN

There is no one who hasn't experienced some sort of flareup, acid skin burn, excessive oil and/or facial flushing at one time or another, from blushing in response to an emotional encounter to a zit before the "prom." Oriental diagnosis views a pimple on your chin as a possible indication of mental stress, and many dermatologists and estheticians, as well, have noted the emotional link. This happens to some skins on a regular basis. It just seems that some people have emotionally sensitive skin. See also *Acne Rosacea.*

SPECIAL CARE

OverSeasoned Sensitive skins should **avoid rough abrasives,** particularly those made of seeds or nuts. Topically apply **vitamin E only if it has been dispersed in another oil** or cream; not all vitamin E is the same and some forms when directly applied to the skin will provoke a sensitive reaction. **Wear rubber gloves** when cleaning. **Don't use paper tissues;** they contain fine wood particles that will scratch and irritate. Opt rather for cotton puffs. **Don't scratch, rub or abrade** or in any way treat your skin harshly. If you've got an itch, "cool" it by placing soothing ice over the problem for a few seconds. If your sensitivities are emotionally linked, **get into the exercise habit**—release a few endorphins. They'll balance your emotional outlook.

RECIPES

COMFORTING COMPOTE

Yogurt, honey, oatmeal, grapes and melon can be particularly soothing to sensitive skins. But always test first!

See also *Recipes for All Occasions*.

OLIVE OILY

Did your ancestors come from olive country—the Mediterranean or the Middle East? Your skin is, more than likely, **Olive Oily.** Oily skin is genetic, and dark haired olive complexions are typically, though not necessarily, oily. Visible pores keep skin oily to the touch and the forehead and chin look shiny. Unless pores are conscientiously cared for, even in adulthood, clogging can result in acne, blemishes and scarring. Properly cared for, oily skin can be blemish free.

The excess oil is the result of overactive sebaceous glands that are directly linked by hormonal activity. Overproduction of sebum is experienced by most of us in adolescence. It is also noted by women prior to menstruation, and some women may notice a decrease in oil production during the last half of pregnancy, with a speed up just after giving birth and then back to normal.

Seasonal changes, sex and age affect oil production. Hot oily perspiration in summer opposes a drier cold winter condition. In adulthood, men produce more sebum than women. With age, hormonal production slows, and oil production slows along with it. Women note a sharp decline after menopause, while a man's oil production slackens in the sixties.

The good news is that your skin will remain smooth and moist as you age and there will be fewer zits and pimples to contend with. Protected against moisture loss and dryness, Olive Oily skins will shun the tiny lines and wrinkles associated with drier skins.

DIETARY HELP

If your skin is excessively oily, it may indicate a lack of vitamins B2 or B6. See *The Skin-Vites*. If you are prone to "breakouts," cutting down your daily consumption of fats and oils and androgen producing foods may be worth consideration. See *Potluck Acne, Dietary Help*.

SPECIAL CARE

Steer clear of pore clogging heavy creams and moisturizers. Choose, rather, a humectant such as **aloe, glycerin or honey, and emollients of cold pressed vegetable oil.** If you purchase cosmetics, be sure they are noncomedegeneic, i.e. do not have a tendency to clog pores. Choose **water-based foundations.** Mild scrubs are fine used two or three times weekly. They deep clean, but will also activate your already overactive sebaceous glands. Close your pores with a **vodka, alcohol or lemon astringent-toner.**

Oily skins need to use an astringent-toner that contains alcohol, **witch hazel** and/or citrus extracts. They will absorb excess oil (a bacterial breeding ground) and kill the bacteria. Use them only on oily areas. After washing your face, saturate a cotton ball or pad and wipe it gently over the oily areas once or twice a day. If your astringent is causing redness on the oily areas of your face, it is too strong. You may wish to try lemon juice cut with aloe juice or floral waters.

RECIPES

BREWER'S YEAST MASKS

Periodic face masks with brewer's yeast can help control an Olive Oily complexion. A plain mask of just brewer's yeast and water will do fine, or see The Youthful Yeast Yummy.

CLAY, FRUITS AND VEGETABLE MASKS

A clay mask of kaolin or fuller's earth moistened with cabbage juice, left on the skin for twenty minutes, is excellent for oily skin.

Instead of cabbage juice, you might choose mashed strawberries, grapes, lemon or lemon juice or pear, and a drop or two of the essential oils Frankincense and Camphor—among others they have a balancing effect. (Leave on for 20 minutes). Rinse.

For more helpful hints see *PotLuck Acne; Recipes for All Occasions* and *Gourmet Ingredients.*

CHEF'S T-ZONE COMBO

Just because the **Chef's T-Zone Combo** is, by far, the most common skin type, doesn't mean it is the most easily handled. In fact, it can be very tricky. If you are a Chef's T-Zone Combo, you might have two faces in one, combining Olive Oily visible pores and oil across the forehead, on the bridge of the nose, on the nose, at the sides of the nose and the chin, in what is called the "T-Zone," while your cheeks can be Regular Tossed Normal to Crouton Dry.

Combination skin can be mild, seeming almost normal. Or it can be extreme, when pores in the T-Zone are quite large, excessively oily, clogged and erupted, while the cheek area is reminiscent of the Sahara. To add to the complexity, some areas within the T-Zone may be oiler than others.

And, just to keep you on your toes, your Chef's T-Zone Combo can subtly change in degrees of oiliness and dryness, so your daily skin care regimen will have to change with it. Diet will affect your skin; stress, hormonal cycles, and overnight cold snaps and weather changes can make a difference.

Extreme combinations must be treated as both oily and dry. If you are an Extreme Chef's T-Zone combo, take great care with the products you choose so as not to further aggravate either condition. Read both *Crouton Dry* and *Olive Oily* for hints on skin care. Also you may wish to include *Pot-Luck Acne* and/or *Marinading Mature*.

POTLUCK ACNE

Potluck Acne is a chronic skin condition in which overactivity of the sebaceous glands combines with bacterial infection. Too much sebum (oil) pours onto the skin's surface, mixes with environmental dirt and dead skin cells which are as a matter of course flaking off the skin's surface. This unhappy mix becomes a bacterial breeding ground where pores become blocked, blackheads form, congested hair follicles become infected and the liquid that seeps from the infected areas infects the surrounding tissue.

WHY ACNE?

Why acne happens to some skins and not others, all factors seemingly equal, is still a mystery. Genetic predisposition is involved. Some skins just don't seem to slough off the dead skin cells that wrap around from the surface into the opening of the sebaceous follicular canal (pore) as efficiently as others and so, the pore becomes blocked. (See *illustration* next page). If you have one or two pimples, you do not necessarily have acne; but if you repeatedly have comedones you may have a mild case.

Affecting almost 80 percent of all teenagers, according to some figures, **acne vulgaris** is the most common form of acne. Although most cases of adolescent acne are usually mild, true acne may sometimes linger until the forties, some cases beginning long after the teens. **Acne conglobata** is more severe,

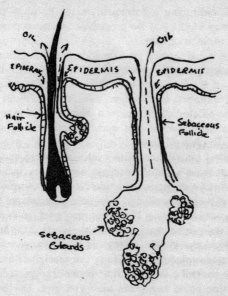

affecting more men than women, occurring, usually, between the ages of 18 and 30. It can come and go for years. There is still a more serious form that is very rare and can be accompanied by fever, swollen joints and anemia. Yet, by classification, acne is acne. There is no special term to differentiate a mild case from a severe one. However, not all acne is alike, so acne is graded from one to four depending on the extent and severity, acne conglobata being listed in grade four.

THE HORMONE-OIL-STRESS CONNECTION

No one knows for sure what causes acne, but there is a definite tie between excessive oil, stress and hormone production, even though dry skin can suffer from acne as well. Not everyone with oily skin will have acne, however, nor will everyone undergoing a hormonal change or stress incur an acne flareup. But if you are predisposed to the condition, the odds are in favor of acne.

Both men and women produce androgens (male hormones) and estrogen (female hormones), the sexual balance being in the ratio of the hormones to each other. During puberty, the powerful androgen, testosterone, formed in the testes in men and in the ovaries and adrenals in women, is in excess. This triggers a chain reaction that stimulates the sebaceous glands to increased oil production.

In adults, natural hormonal cycles and fluctuations, also stress, can cause a similar reaction. Anytime the male-female **hormone ratio changes,** as in adolescence, menstrual fluctuations and pregnancy swings, then acne flare-ups are likely.

Stress can cause acne. Periods of fear, grief, anticipation of an event, daily pressures, even extreme joy, affect the hormone-producing adrenal glands. All register as stress to your adrenals.

Hormone replacement therapy can precipitate acne. Taking **birth control pills** or quitting them can trigger acne problems lasting up to two years after you quit. The first birth control pills on the market some 30 years ago were high in estrogens and many cases of acne improved with the taking. Some of the side effects of estrogens were less than desirable, however, and the amounts of estrogen in the pills, along with their acne relieving potential, have been greatly reduced. In fact, some of the newer formulations will aggravate acne. Birth control pills also tend to deplete the body of some of the B-vitamins which are necessary for healthy skin; this can cause problems. If you are taking birth control pills, be sure to supplement with the entire B-complex. *Birth control pills that aggravate acne include Norinyl, Norlestrin, Ortho-Novum and Ovral. Those that help clear include Enovid-E, Enovid-5, Demulen and Ovulen.*

Although excessive oil production is a contributing factor, some researchers are questioning testosterone sensitivity as the underlying cause of acne.

OTHER CAUSES

Rubbing, pressing, abrading and irritating the skin by any "mechanical" means, whether it's with a buff puff or from leaning on your own hands. Sleeping on your face or pressing into the telephone speaker can also produce bumps or **acne mechanica.** Closely allied to this is **clothing acne** where irritation can result from your favorite wool sweater or perspiration combined with synthetic fabric sensitivity.

Using cosmetics that are too oily for your skin, can cause **cosmetic or makeup acne.** When looking for makeup, choose noncomedegeneic, or non–pore clogging, formulations. They are usually oil-free.

Fluoride acne can cause irritated mouth corners, encourage zits around the mouth and chin and redden faces from under the nose down.

For some people just living in the tropics can cause **tropical acne** that disappears when moving to a cooler climate.

Sun-induced acne, also called **Caribbean** or **Mallorca acne** (in Europe) can be caused by the sun itself, or a combination of sun and **sunscreen ingredients.** This acne type can be seen 8–10 weeks after exposure to the sun. Your tan already faded, tiny little pustules appear, usually on the back and shoulders.

Animals fed steroids similar to androgens whose meat is eaten can cause **food acne.** Milk, high in progesterone, can cause difficulties. Other problem foods are: wheat germ, peanuts, liver, kidney and organ meats and gluten in bread and wheat products. Cooking over a greasy splattering pan can also cause acne.

Iodide acne can result from eating artichokes, spinach, kelp and seaweeds, also, shellfish. Certain soft drinks containing brominated vegetables can result in **bromide acne.**

Asthma and cold sufferers can be the acne victims of bromides and iodides in their medications. **Medication acne** can affect people on barbiturates—sleeping pills that contain barbiturates can precipitate or aggravate acne, and cause ''a fixed drug eruption'' in which a red or purple lesion appears each time the drug is taken and leaves a permanent brown discoloration. Tranquilizers, hormone therapy (Danazol-synthetic androgen to treat endometriosis; also, steroids), lithium, and drugs that treat epilepsy (Phenytoin), tuberculosis (INH), among others, can also precipitate problems.

Other acnes can be provoked by **headbands or sweatbands;** backpacks; **makeup and hair cosmetics** that get caught in the hairline; hair worn over the face in bangs; industrial compounds—such as coal tars and chlorinated hydrocarbons; **certain vitamins in excess**—*B12, particularly in injections, can cause acne flare-ups, also vitamin E and multivitamin/mineral supplements, especially the iodides usually taken by pregnant women.* However, a **deficiency of vitamin B2 or B6** can increase oiliness. Many factors can trigger acne. It may be up to you to track down the precipitating villains.

SOME ACNE TERMS

A comedone is a clogged pore. Filled with sebum, dead skin cells and bacteria, it may appear as a whitehead (closed comedone) or a blackhead (open comedone).

A blackhead is called open, because it is visible to the eye and is easily recognized due to the dark oxidation of the dried sebum.

A closed comedone, or whitehead, is shiny, pale and slightly elevated, so tiny it can better be felt than seen. It will either erupt to form a blackhead, or inflame causing a pimple known to dermatologists as either . . .

a papule (a tiny inflamed pimple) that can totally clear spontaneously in about two or three weeks. Or . . .

a pustule, a larger inflamed pus-filled pimple that, if superficial, will begin to clear in a couple of days leaving no scars. **Severe pustules,** however, may take up to six weeks to clear, and often leave scars. A larger, deep-seated pustule is a . . .

nodule. Sometimes called **cystic acne,** this acne-type lesion is more inflamed than a pustule, can be very painful and can scar. **Cysts** are more deeply imbedded and are the most painful of the acne lesions.

HERBAL BALANCERS

Adolescent boys and young men often clear acne with the herbal *combination of Sarsaparilla and Siberian Ginseng,* male hormone balancers, taken as tea or in capsules.

The following are **female herbal balancers,** usually used in combination and easily found ready prepared in extracts or capsules. They can be found in health food stores or ordered through herb houses. Combinations can be alternated.

Combo 1. *Golden Seal, Red Raspberry Leaves, Black Cohosh, Queen of the Meadow, Marshmallow Root, Blessed Thistle, Lobelia, Capsicum, Ginger, Dong Quoi (also known as Tang-kuei or Angelica root).*

Combo 2. *Herbal combination traditionally used for women who can't take estrogen are Golden Seal, Capsicum, False Unicorn Root, Ginger, Uva Ursi Leaves, Cramp Bark, Squaw Vine, Blessed Thistle, Red Raspberry leaves.*

Herbal hormone **balancers for both sexes** include these combinations:

Combo 1. *Siberian Ginseng Root, Echinacea Root, Saw Palmetto Berries, Gotu Kola, Damiana Leaves, Sarsaparilla, Periwinkle, Garlic, Capsicum, Chickweed.*

Combo 2. *Black Cohosh, Licorice, False Unicorn, Siberian Ginseng, Sarsaparilla, Squaw Vine, Blessed Thistle.*

If acne responds to antibiotics, **strong scented garlic capsules** may also work. *Garlic is a natural antibiotic that also contains hormones.*

DIETARY HELP

Should I or shouldn't I? Will it or won't it? The food-acne connection theories bounce back and forth. Until recently, the theory was that you could eat anything and it wouldn't affect acne or your oil production one way or the other. Common sense prevailing, the thinking now is that it does. If a pimple shows up pretty regularly after a chocolate binge or french fried onion rings make a note to adjust your menu.

As mentioned, some of the most likely **acne provoking foods** *include milk and dairy products. High in progesterone and high on food sensitivity lists, milk and dairy products are also high in fats. Avoiding dairy products for about a month, then gauging your reaction as you reintroduce one item at a time might be a thought.*

Other indictable foods include: wheat germ: peanuts (that includes peanut butter or wheat germ bread); salted nuts; crackers (many are deep fried); shellfish (freshwater fish is best) and foods high in iodine, kelp, artichokes and spinach (high in halogen); beef, kidney, liver, and other organ meats (high in androgens); caffeine (chocolate, coffee, colas) and alcohol.

Helpful: Supplements of Vitamin A; 10,000IU–20,000IU daily including a multivitamin supplement; Zinc 50mg on top of your multivite; amino acid—L-lysine 500 mg daily are sometimes recommended. Also, increased intake of unsaturated fatty acids (vitamin F) in the form of wheat germ, or wheat germ oil; sunflower and safflower oils are also high in unsaturated fatty acids.

SPECIAL CARE

Cleanse your face two or three times a day. Mild scrubs are fine used two or three times weekly. They deep clean, but will also activate your already overactive sebaceous glands.

Use an astringent, which is a toner that contains alcohol, witch hazel and/or citrus extracts. The purpose being the absorption of excess oil (a bacterial breeding ground) and to kill the bacteria. The **astringent is to be used on oily areas only;** after washing your face, saturate a cotton ball or pad and wipe it gently over the oily areas once or twice a day. If your astringent causes redness to the oily areas of your face, your astringent is too strong. You may prefer lemon juice diluted with floral or herbal waters. See *Resurrection Dressings.*

Steer clear of pore clogging heavy creams and moisturizers. Best bets *include humectants such as aloe or honey-containing "recipes."* Contrary to what many might think, *cold pressed vegetable oils as moisturizers do not clog pores or aggravate acne. They are absorbed slightly into the upper layer of the skin.* **Avoid vasolines and mineral, also baby oil** which is the same thing, a petroleum by-product. If you purchase cosmetics, be sure they are **noncomedegeneic,** i.e., do not have a tendency to clog pores. Choose **water-based foundations.**

Exercise to relieve stress and help rebalance your hormonal levels. *Be sure to start with a clean face* to avoid aggravating your condition with dirt and/or makeup mixed with skin oils and perspiration. *Cleanse after exercising,* as well.

RECIPES

ALOE ADE

Aloe is a wonderful body cleanser. Topically applied, it has helped clear acne. It also has been known to help from the inside when taken as follows: 3 oz. in 8 oz. glass of water, 3 times a day for 10 days, then 2 oz. twice daily for one month. Continue until definite improvement is noted, then reduce aloe to one ounce 2 times a day until acne is cleared. For regular daily use, see also *Skin Juices*. Note cautions if diabetic.

LEMON AID

Wash or pat your face with lemon three times a day.

GARLIC GALA

Put a clove of garlic into a garlic press, and dab onto blemishes to dry. Garlic is also antibiotic.

IDAHO A-GO-GO

Otherwise know as the potato pat. *Dab the juice of a raw "Idaho" on your blemishes.*

THE YOLKS ON YOU

Not too long ago, the following recipe for acne blemishes was printed in the Ann Landers column. Then, quite by accident, a lady who had mistaken Anti-Aging Press for a cosmetic company, called from across the country and, in conversation, told me that she, too, had tried it and it really worked, even on her arms. *Simply apply raw egg yolk (high in sulphur and vitamin A) to your skin. Allow to dry for 10 minutes. Rinse well. Repeat daily for one month. By then the blemishes should be gone. Repeat the application twice a month for three months. If troubled again, repeat applications.*

LEMON-EGG DROP

For a mask that cuts oil while tightening pores, *mix together an egg white with lemon juice. Using a cosmetic brush, paint your face with the mixture. Allow to dry. Rinse with warm water.* Especially good in the T-Zone.

FREEZING OUT THE ZITS

Cold treatments help put the chill on acne. Lesions dry faster. See: *Fresh from the Crisper.* Bonus: You'll get a face lift, to boot!

STEAMING OUT THE ZITS

Strawberry Leaves, Red Clover and Lavender Leaves in a facial sauna are antiseptic and stimulate new tissue growth. Or try 5 drops of one or a blend of the following essential oils: Lavender, Cedarwood, Sweet Thyme.

BLOTTING UP THE ZITS

A clay mask (kaolin or fuller's earth) moistened with cabbage juice is excellent for oily skin (Leave on for 20 minutes). Substitutes for cabbage juice, or used in combination with, are grape and/or tomato, and one or two or a blend of the following essences Camphor, Juniper, Bergamot (2 or 3 drops). A little brewer's yeast may also be added.

Periodic face masks with brewer's yeast have been known to help. See *The Youthful Yeast Yummy*—as blemishes clear, sagging skin tightens.

PRESSING OUT THE ZITS

If you are going to try to remove your own blackheads or "pop" your own pimples, and we all do, never, never use your bare fingers and especially not your nails. You can work with tissue wrapped around your fingers or with cotton swabs.

Blackheads. The best time to attempt to tackle a blackhead according to most skin care experts is after a facial that has included steaming. If you haven't steamed for about 15 minutes, be sure to apply a warm softening compress first. While your skin is still soft and pores are still open, the extracting can begin.

   Standing in front of a brightly lit mirror, tissues or cotton swabs in place, press gently around the base of the blackhead with an upward, outward movement. If unsuccessful with your first try, pause several seconds, then try again. If still unsuccessful, don't force the issue, irritation could result in an infection.

Pimples are not nearly as difficult to remove as blackheads, but timing is everything. Do not attempt until you see the whites of their heads! At this time, press a hot compress over the pimple to soften the area. Proceed as above. It may take more than one try to remove all the pus. But, take care, do not irritate the area.

When finished, an alcohol-based astringent will disinfect *all skin types*. Most skin care experts agree that you should not attempt a full face extraction more than once a week. If you have a good esthetician, it is best to give him or her the job.

ACNE ROSACEA

An acnelike condition, **acne rosacea** is very different from ordinary "garden variety" acne. There is excessive redness in the cheeks and nose, greasiness, enlarged pores, lumpy swellings, thick skin and often permanent scarring. Sometimes a staph infection is also involved.

Aggravated by emotions, rosy, fair, thin-skinned women with tempers are excellent candidates for rosacea. Most often incurred by women, it tends to be more serious in men. Rare in youth, rosacea *develops over a period of years,* appearing, at first, as a *temporary flush in the center of the face.* The result of vasodilation (the expansion of small blood vessels), rosacea is different from a blush, distinguished by its intensity and duration. Whether temporary or almost permanent, the flush eventually encompasses the cheeks and chin, broken blood vessels showing up at the sides of the nose. *Suppressing emotions, such as fear and anger, will increase the occurrences, as will the anticipation of important events or unpleasant scenes.* This also increases the damaging potential to the skin. After dilating repeatedly, the blood vessels lose the ability to shrink and the face remains flushed.

Rosacea, like acne, is not fully understood. Often, it is accompanied by dandruff, as well as oily skin and pimples, particularly on the nose. When severe, rosacea can redden eyelids and affect the mucous membranes of the eye causing conjunctivitis. Eyes that burn and sting often accompany the flushed, blotchy, highly strung, intense victims of rosacea, who are, many times, mistaken for heavy drinkers.

DIETARY HELP

Rosacea-prone skins seem to be affected by foods and especially, the **temperature of foods** that dilate the capillaries. Sipping cool water or iced drinks with a hot meal may help avoid the flush. **Steer clear of refined carbohydrates:** sugar, candy, pastries, also capillary dilating **spicy foods,** which, on the whole, may not be as detrimental as the temperature, but also include mustard, catsup and relishes.

Histamines (chemicals found naturally in the body, and in some plants and animals) and **tyramine** have been cited as the worst offenders. Histamines are contained in red wine and beer, champagne, bourbon, gin and vodka (white wine is okay).

Aged cheeses contain tyramine. Definitely no cheddar and camembert. Cottage cheese is okay. Avoid **fermented, pickled, and smoked food.** Hold the **MSG** in Chinese takeout, also the hot spices and **soy sauce.** (*Read labels, many prepared foods contain MSG.*) No **hot dogs** at the ball park, or after-the-game **cold cuts,** salami, pepperoni and other hard sausages, and don't bring home the **bacon**—all contain nitrates).

Organ meats, especially liver, and yeast extract are no-nos. So are **sour fruits or veggies, especially citrus, pineapples, and tomatoes. Watch out for bananas, figs, avocados, peppers, raisins, nuts, vanilla extract, coffee, tea and colas.** When supplementing with vitamins, avoid the **niacin**-flush—large doses of B3, which cause blood to flood to the skin's surface. *Small 10 mg doses of Riboflavin (B2), twice daily, may help.*

Giving up on your diet? Don't! Start step by step. Customize. Experts suggest eating bland cool foods and building from there. Try a cold potato or a cold turnip and start adding in and trying foods, gauging your reactions as you go.

SPECIAL CARE

Your skin is sensitive, so treat it very gently. Do not use scrubs or mechanical exfoliants of any kind (including a wash-cloth); avoid very hot (this includes steaming, hot tubs and saunas) and very cold water. Stay out of the sun. Use a sun-screen. Avoid getting overheated. Read cosmetic labels, sorbic acid in some formulations will cause vasodilation.

Exercise is important *for rosacea complexions. Exercises that cause you to overheat, however, should not be undertaken. Swimming in cool water is great. Easy bicycling. Yoga and relaxing meditation could help you to release those minor ir-ritations that can destroy your skin.*

RECIPES

The following can also help: dressings and masks that con-tain Aloe Vera, Ginseng, Squalene, Rosehips and Chamomile. Very helpful is the essential oil Blue Chamomile (German Chamomile). Very high in Azulene (actually, Chamazulen) and Bisabolol, it is very soothing on severe inflammations. Also Tea Tree Oil can be safely dabbed full strength on painful pimples, reducing the heat and inflammation. See also *Mois-turizing Mists; Exotic Marinades; Gourmet Ingredients; Masques Exotique.*

Your dermatologist may have other ideas as well. Check with him before starting your at-home help. Estrogen is some-times prescribed for postmenopausal rosacea complexions. See also *Herbal Balancers,* pages 65–6.

FRIDGEWORN DEVITALIZED

FridgeWorn Devitalized can describe a basically *healthy skin that is fatigued*. It can reflect the *result of prolonged mental, emotional or physical stress, illness, exhaustion, lack of sleep, overwork, food or drug abuse*. Depleted skin is lacking life, zip, zest, and the glow of healthy red corpuscles perking through robust capillaries. Many times, more easily identified than corrected, FridgeWorn Devitalized *may be the direct result of life-style, compulsions, or ingrained habits*.

Excess caffeine, found in coffee, chocolate, tea, cocoa and cola drinks can deplete skin of B-vitamins, calcium and iron. Dependency on diuretics and laxatives, alcohol and drug abuse, or starvation diets can devitalize by washing vital minerals, vitamins and nutrients out of your system and prevent them from being properly assimilated.

A **smoker's face,** most commonly associated with Fridge-Worn, is not only devitalized but is toxic from the smoke. In fact, if you live with or are regularly in the proximity of a heavy smoker, your face will also show the effects. Deficient in oxygen and nutrients, a ''smoker's face'' has been identified as having one or more of the following characteristics: crow's feet from squinting, gauntness, a leathery rugged appearance, a slight pigmented gray tone, bags and dark circles under the eyes and pucker lines around the lips from puffing. Depriving your skin of its normal blood flow, you are actually starving your skin and, after thirty, aging your face twice as fast as that of a non-smoker. Smoking depletes vitamins A, B-complex, C and E, as well as minerals: calcium, potassium and zinc, not only from your skin, but from your entire system.

DIETARY HELP

If a life-style or a detrimental habit is causing your face to deteriorate, you must first decide if your face is worth the effort to make the life-style change. While you are deciding, there is a wealth of nutritional information available to help counter the effects. For instance, a smoker would, according to research, supplement with large doses of vitamin C and beta carotene, as well as some vitamin E, all free-radical fighters to help replace what is going up in smoke and to prevent cross-linking of damaged cells. There are programs to help smokers and substance abusers whose faces will ultimately reflect the effects of nutritional imbalances. Workaholics are also at risk, and yo-yo dieters can literally wear out their faces from years of losing and gaining, gaining and losing, until their facial "elastic" is shot.

Your skin is, after all, the reflection of the total you. Think adequate nutrition, fresh raw fruits and vegetables, protein, complex carbs, plenty of water and rest, a gentle balanced exercise program and a good vitamin-mineral supplement.

If you are devitalized from the flu or a week long marathon, your entire body needs to be rebalanced. Take a good look at the *Skin Juices* in the beginning of the book. They can help you jump start, "crisping your leaves" in a hurry. The carrot-celery combo is an excellent traditional recipe for revitalizing after illness or exhaustion; also, the **raw potassium broth** made of the raw freshly juiced carrots, celery, parsley, potatoes and spinach. Organic minerals and salts in this "broth" encompass almost the entire range needed by the body. Go easy on the parsley, however, it is very powerful.

Devitalized skin may be suffering from anemia. An excellent iron tonic that does wonders is made by **Floridex.** Made totally from plant and herbal sources, it is readily assimilated. Iron-rich foods include parsley, raisins, squash, kidneys, liver, split peas, beans, carrots, spinach, lean red meat, pork, lamb, shellfish, chicken and turkey (dark meat) and eggs.

RECIPES

THE HON-"E" PAT

Pierce and squeeze a vitamin E capsule into 2 teaspoons of honey. Mix. Pat all over your face and neck. Marinate for about 20 minutes. Great for saggy devitalized skin in need of moisture and nutrition.

CARROT-OATMEAL MASH-QUE

1 cup cooked oatmeal, slightly warm
2–4 drops of Carrot Seed oil (See *Gourmet Ingredients*)

Mix. Apply to your face and neck for 20 minutes. Rinse. Apply moisturizer. See also *Dressings for all Occasions*.

OVERRIPE FRUIT

Do you feel like an **OverRipe Fruit** whose seeds are ready to burst and sprout? The water balance in your body is off. Just as dehydrated skin can result from a lack of fluid intake, too much moisture will result in a watery complexion. This doesn't usually mean that you are drinking too much water, but, rather, that your fluid removing mechanism isn't functioning properly. Overhydrated skin is most likely caused by diet, but persistent edema should be addressed by your doctor just on the off-chance that it may be caused by a kidney, bladder, heart or liver infection, inflammation or malfunction. Usually noted in the feet and ankles, any part of the body can be edemic.

DIETARY HELP

If your complexion is watery, **"think salt."** Edema or fluid retention may be the result of excessive salt in the diet. Some foods that bring salt to mind are: caviar (sorry), bacon, herring, soy sauce, pickles, olives, canned veggies and processed foods, some frozen foods have hidden salt (read labels), shellfish, and bouillon cubes. Fried and smoked foods, white sugar, white flour, chocolate, dairy products (quiche, processed cheeses), duck and sometimes animal protein can encourage water retention, as well as food allergies.

Increase your raw food intake. Include apples, onions, beets and grapes, eggs, broiled white fish and skinless chicken or turkey. Small amounts of cottage cheese, yogurt, buttermilk and kefir are okay.

Supplementing with vitamin C may be helpful. Mildly diuretic, "C" is essential for adrenal function, as well as the production of adrenal hormones vital for your fluid balance. Also useful in edema: Horsetail, Juniper Berries, Pau d'arco, Cornsilk, Kelp, Marshmallow, Parsley and Dandelion Root.

SPECIAL CARE

Exercise is important for circulation and the elimination of excess fluids. **Exercise daily. Consider hot baths and/or saunas twice a week. Avoid stress.**

RECIPE IDEA

A facial mask of clay or oatmeal with the addition of the essential oils of Lavender and/or Juniper will help to dehydrate. Other helpful oils include: Eucalyptus, Sage, Cypress, Fennel, Geranium, Rosemary and Patchouli. Do not leave on longer than 20 minutes. Wash off thoroughly with warm water. See *Masques Exotique* for proper proportions.

MARINADING MATURE

Some of the best "cooking," the most fun, and the most astounding changes can result in **Marinading Mature** skin. So, if you are over thirty-five, feel you are slowing down and are noticing uncomfortable *signs of the times:* some sagging, brown spots and the "R" word—*wrinkles,* stay confident. We can smooth out the problems together, whatever they are, or at the very least, make noticeable improvements.

Before we start, it might be a good idea to get the "lay of the lettuce," so to speak. If you know what's going on, you can not only counter the effects, but some of the causes as well.

TRUE AGING VERSUS PHOTOAGING

There are two types of skin aging. One is **true aging.** This happens very, very slowly, as long as you take good care of yourself. Eat well. Supplement with needed protein, vitamins, minerals, hormones and enzymes. Sleep well, exercise and relax well. Drink plenty of "well" (i.e., healthy) water. Keep busy, think positive and have a dream to fulfill. It also helps to love well, notice I didn't say wisely, just well. If you do all this, there's no reason why you shouldn't age well, or rather stay young and vital for a long long time. To date, no one has conquered death and taxes, but we have learned that we can slow down the so called *aging process,* and certainly a great deal can be done to keep our skin taut, blemish and wrinkle-free.

Oh yes, and screen well—definitely wear a sunscreen. Because the other type of skin aging is **photoaging**. *It is, in fact, the most dramatic type of aging, causing most of the negative effects that we associate with ancient skin—and* **photoaging can be totally prevented.** See *The ''R'' Word: ''Wrinkles.''*

COUNTERING TRUE AGING

True aging produces some definite changes in the skin. But, you can help to a great extent to counter your slowdown. Listed here are some causes, effects and countermeasures.

THE SITUATION

Dry skin is almost synonymous with mature complexions. All skin thins, loses moisture and oil with time. The oil glands that gave you so much trouble as a teenager started to slow down in your twenties along with moisture-laden perspiration. The mucopolysaccharides (natural humectants), and particularly hyaluronic acid, that hold moisture to the skin have also declined.

If you had normal skin as a teenager, you will be using fairly heavy moisturizers by the time you're fifty. If you had excessively oily skin in adolescence, then 50 will be your time to *shine* in an entirely different way—your skin will definitely have an edge on moisture; it will wrinkle less and later. Generally, the darker a complexion, the oilier the skin, and a bonus—it is also thicker and able to hold moisture more effectively. Another plus, darker skin contains more melanin, the pigment that gives it color and offers protection from the sun. So, darker, oilier complexions may do more suffering in puberty, but stand a better chance of aging gracefully with less help.

THE COUNTERMEASURES

Moisturize from the inside, see *Succulent Seductive Skin* and *The Skin Juices*. See also *Dietary Help* for Marinading Mature skin with particular focus on digestive enzymes. And, moisturize from the outside—mucopolysaccharide-containing aloe can be a lifesaver, also hydrating honey masks and lactic acid-containing buttermilk. See *Crouton Dry* for tips, also *Exotic Marinades* (solutions from aromatheraphy) and *Monday Marinades* (intensive care formulas). Avoid drying astringent-toners with alcohol, witch hazel or citrus extracts that absorb excess oil or use them only on overly oily areas of your face.

THE SITUATION

With age the skin's ability to heal and repair itself is less effective. Collagen, the skin's "cement," becomes cross-linked and degenerates with age. *Free radical cross-linking in the skin, caused by environmental pollutants, UV radiation and unhealthy living habits, occurs when sugar molecules (glucose) bind skin proteins stiffening the protein fibers resulting in degeneration.*

THE COUNTERMEASURES

Supplement with free radical fighting vitamins A, C, and E to retard or prevent cross-linking. Eat foods rich in enzyme SOD (superoxide dismutase), known also to lighten brown age spots. It is found in yeast and potato skins; (See *The Youthful Yeast Yummy*). Include zinc (promotes wound healing), gamma-linoleic acid (GLA), and free form amino acids, particularly L-cystine that aids in the formation of the skin, l-lysine, and l-glutathione. Check into Pycnogenol (pick-**na**-gen-ol), a patented bioflavonoid blend that is super-oxidant. It is 50 times more powerful than vitamin E and 20 times greater than "C." See also *Plant Food Plus,* and *Exotic Marinades* for essential oils that promote tissue regeneration and increase cell turnover. Include these, along with the vitamin "A-C-Es" in your daily skin recipes. Also, see *The "R" Word: "Wrinkles"* and *Anti-Aging Antioxidants*.

THE SITUATION

Your skin's lower layer, the dermis, becomes thinner and blood vessels in the skin decrease with the accompanying decrease in circulation. This means less oxygen and nutrition is getting to the skin.

THE COUNTERMEASURES
Exercise. Twenty minutes a day, 5 days a week of **aerobic activity,** not only increases circulation, strengthens the heart, bone and muscles, increases oxygenation of the blood and the body, but has been shown to increase the thickness of the skin. Also, improve your blood and oxygen with the following deep breathing exercise: for one month, hold your breath for thirty seconds every half hour.

Feed your skin from the outside as well as the inside. Your skin is a two-way suit that will absorb nutrition. Since it is the farthest away from the body's food source, it only makes sense to feed it from the outside as well. Aloe, for instance, penetrates all skin layers and can help transport other vitamins and nutrients from the outside in. Rejuvenating essential oils very effectively penetrate all layers as well. See *Recipes for All Occasions*.

THE SITUATION

As skin ages, the number of ultraviolet shielding melanocytes (cells that produce melanin) diminish.

THE COUNTERMEASURE
Sunscreen. See also *The "R" Word: "Wrinkles."*

THE SITUATION

With time, the rate of epidermal cell replacement slows down. From age 30 to 80 the rate of cell turnover can diminish up to 50 percent.

THE COUNTERMEASURES

Exfoliate. Removing the dead upper layer encourages cell turnover in the basal (lower dermis) layer. Also speed up cell turnover with essential oils. See *Scrub Those Carrots, Peel Those Potatoes; Wilted Salad Supreme; Exotic Marinades; and Gourmet Ingredients.*

Make sure you **get enough deep "beauty" sleep.** The human growth hormone is released when you sleep. These hormones may have skin specific relatives that speed up the production of collagen.

THE SITUATION

Langerhans' cells (immune cells) in the skin are greatly reduced with age; the skin has less ability to reduce infections.

THE COUNTERMEASURES

Supplement with immune strengthening nutrients. See Dietary Help for Marinading Mature skin. Bathe in immune strengthening essential oils, such as Lavender; use them in your everyday recipes. See *Exotic Marinades.* Watch your diet more carefully. Avoid refined foods, sugar, grains. Be sure to include cleansing fiber to scrub out internal toxins that weaken the body. Drink sufficient water and juices. Include enzymes, exercise, and proper rest. Topical application of the vitamins A-C-E can benefit. See also *The Skin-Vites.*

THE SITUATION

A yellow pigment, lipofuscin, will sometimes accumulate in the dermis causing a **yellow appearance** in aging tissue.

THE COUNTERMEASURE

Vitamin E taken orally will, many times counteract the condition.

THE SITUATION

As the skin ages, there is a **flattening out of the basement layer** (the tissue that joins the upper epidermis and the lower dermis). Since the layers of the skin are not as tightly bound, transfer of nutrients and information between the two layers is reduced. Elastin fibers become thicker, less springy. Enzymes necessary for collagen stabilization decline.

THE COUNTERMEASURES

Aerobic exercise increases the flow of oxygen and nutrition. Also, stimulate and regenerate with **finger pressure massage** techniques, shiatsu or acupressure on the facial points, as well as the skin-toning body points, as in **Facelift Naturally.**

Look into supplementation with vitamins, minerals, enzymes, and other hormone balancing herbs, such as, ginseng for men and women, as well as using essential oils that penetrate into your skin's basement layer facilitating regeneration of the dermal cells. **Feed your skin with vitamins, minerals and enzymes in nourishing masks, dressing and marinades, from without as well as within.**

THE SITUATION

Soluble collagen decreases and insoluble collagen increases. The skin becomes less pliant.

THE COUNTERMEASURES

Aloe applied topically to the skin of laboratory animals has been shown to increase the soluble collagen. See also the regeneration effects of essential oils in *Exotic Marinades*.

OTHER SIGNS OF THE TIMES

THE SITUATION

Broken Capillaries. Not only associated with mature skin, "broken capillaries" are actually the result of permanently dilated tiny blood vessels close to the surface of the skin. Usually first noticed around the nose, they are most readily visible in thin, transparent skin. No one knows the reason for their appearance though heredity seems to be an important factor. High estrogen levels can increase their number. In some women "small red lines" may first appear in the second to fifth month of pregnancy or when using birth control pills.

However, telangiectases, as they are called, are not strictly a woman's problem. Trauma, even a minor one, just blowing your nose can result in "broken caps." Rough handling of the skin or squeezing the area around the nose may cause an isolated case. Prolonged use of steroid creams, sun damage, hyperthyroidism can all contribute. A male friend in his twenties noticed broken capillaries around his eyes after a niacin flush.

Over-forty women, especially those who have been active outdoors, can be seen with brownish symmetrical netlike broken capillaries on their faces, necks and upper chests in areas that have been exposed to the sun. The areas also become very thin with noticeable hair follicles. Possibly brought on by a hormone-ultraviolet combination, the "marks" can be lightened with bleaching agents, such as lemon and yogurt. Be sure to use sunscreen.

THE COUNTERMEASURES

If you have a tendency to broken capillaries, **avoid** the dilating effects of **alcoholic beverages.** Don't use **harsh grainy scrubs, wash cloths or buff puffs. Avoid pressing, tugging and resting your face in your hands.** Never use **very hot or very cold water,** or go to temperature extremes such as taking a cold shower after exercise, the change is too drastic for your delicate skin. Also, **avoid prolonged exposure to the sun** and don't forget your **sunscreen.**

RECIPE

The following blends of essential oils have been used to repair "broken capillaries":

Blend 1. *Mint, Bay Laurel, Rosemary*
Blend 2. *Chamomile, Parsley and Rose.*
Blend 3. *Cypress and/or Lemon.*

Mix 15 drops of your chosen blend to one ounce of vegetable oil. Gently massage into the broken caps to help restore the natural elasticity of the capillaries. Eventually eliminating the redness, the oils must be massaged faithfully into the skin twice a day for many months before a major improvement is noted, but slight improvement may be noticed after several weeks. See *Exotic Marinades;* also *Gourmet Ingredients* for more information on essential oils. For dietary precautions see *Acne Rosacea.*

THE SITUATION

Brown spots or liver spots develop from about the age of thirty on. Larger than a freckle, flat, oval or round with distinct irregular edges, they appear one at a time, don't fade in winter, and deepen in color. First seen on the face, they will later appear on the hands, wrists and forearms. Most experts agree that they are caused by sun (free radical) damage.

THE COUNTERMEASURES

These marks can be lightened with natural bleaching agents lemon, yogurt, buttermilk, chamomile tea. Topical applications of undiluted aloe have been helpful in hyperpigmentation or liver spots. Finger pressure programs such as **Facelift Naturally** also help lighten.

Damage from free radicals and cross-linking can be greatly diminished by orally taking the vitamins A-C-E, also B1, B5 and B6, bioflavonoids, the minerals zinc and selenium, and the amino acid L-cysteine. (*When taking the B vitamins always include the whole B-complex.*) Remember to wear sunscreen. Even after removal or lightening, sun exposure will cause brown spots to reappear.

THE SITUATION

White Spots or vitiligo. Generally considered a problem of black skin, vitiligo describes a condition where the melancytes just stop working and natural color or skin pigment disappears. Even the fairest skins have pigment, and the condition can occur. It is just more emphasized in darker skins.

THE COUNTERMEASURES

Extra Vitamin C may help, the B-complex taken with extra PABA taken in divided doses throughout the day. Also be sure you are not deficient in HCL (hydrochloric acid), to insure assimilation of the vitamins you are taking. More than a simple C and PABA deficiency, hormonal imbalances and other nutritional imbalances may be involved as well. Wear sunscreen to prevent further damage. See *The Skin Juices* for readily assimilated vitamins and minerals.

DIETARY HELP

Digestive enzymes are important. As one gets older the HCL (hydrochloric acid) naturally found in the stomach diminishes;

without HCL and digestive enzymes, food assimilation is not efficient. You may be eating the most nutritious foods, but if you are not digesting them properly, they cannot be assimilated for skin or body building. Papaya and/or pineapple eaten daily can benefit. They contain enzymes called proteases that can stimulate immune cells and can aid in the destruction of hard bonds, the result of cross-linking, that can cause anything from wrinkles and inflexible arteries to cancer. Consider taking a multidigestive enzyme formula with meals, (if you have ulcers, avoid formulas with HCL).

For healthy skin, a healthy immune system is necessary. Without a healthy immune system, we are susceptible to illness. Illness always shows in the face. Raw thymus glandular stimulates the immune system, as does germanium, vitamins C and A (or beta carotene), and selenium, a powerful antioxidant that works synergistically with vitamin E. Eat high fiber, quality protein, fruits, vegetables, whole grains and nuts.

The B vitamins are very important for healthy skin tone, but many older people have difficulty in assimilating the B's (particularly B12); if this is your case, check with your doctor about vitamin B injections.

Lecithin is necessary for good brain function and for every cell of the body. Unsaturated fatty acids, GLAs, found in vegetable oils are important for cell formation—very high in GLA are: black currant seed oil, evening primrose, borage and salmon oil. A good multivitamin-mineral supplement (*with chelated trace minerals for easier assimilation*) is of value. RNA-DNA is necessary for the production of healthy cells (*do not use if you have a tendency to gout or elevated serum uric acid*). Free form amino acids (*protein supplements*) could be considered, with a small amount of vitamin C and B6 to help assimilation. See also *Plant Food Plus—Feeding Your Skin From Within* and *The "R" Word: "Wrinkles."*

HORMONAL PLANTS AND HERBS

Traditionally herbs, seeds and some everyday seasonings have been used for their hormonal properties. Sage has been used to induce labor, and Fennel to stimulate milk production in lactating animals. Angelica root, known as Tang-kuei (Dong Quoi), has been used for centuries in the orient to balance a woman's problems and Ginseng root a man's. Estrogenic, Ginseng is also taken by menopausal and post menopausal women in teas and capsules.

In the not too distant past, estrogen was given to heart attack prone men with very positive results, but very embarrassing side effects. A traditional remedy for virility and heart problems, it is interesting to note that, although estrogenic, Ginseng also contains testosterone.

Much is still not understood relative to the phytohormones (*plant hormones*). However, listed below are some of the plants that exhibit hormonal characteristics similar to our own. The following are often taken in teas. Many may be added into moisturizing mists or facial splashes. The *dried herbs* are often sprinkled into facial steams and saunas. And *essential oils* may be added into your everyday marinades, dressings, masks and facial steams.

Angelica root, also known as **Tang-kuei (Dong-kwoi),** is estrogenic.

Aniseed. Estrogenic aniseed, also Fennel and Jasmine have been used historically to encourage milk production in lactating or nursing mothers. This is one herb that may be taken in teas, but **never used as the highly concentrated essential oil.** It is highly toxic in this form and addictive. A narcotic that slows the circulation, over time it can damage the brain. *Caution: Never use the essential oil of Anise or Aniseed.*

Chaste tree is a hormone stabilizer.

Eucalyptus is slightly estrogenic.

Fennel (fine in teas and essential oil) is estrogenic.

Garlic contains folliculin, a pre-hormone to estrogen.

Ginseng contains folliculin, testosterone and progesterone.

Hops is estrogenic (folliculin).

Licorice root contains the phytohormone (plant hormone) folliculin. If you have high blood pressure or a kidney disorder, be sure you use the deglycerated form.

Oats contain folliculin.

Sage. The kitchen wouldn't be the same without sage. It is used in cooking, stuffings, for flavoring cheeses. In the past, it has been used in brewing ales and has a very long history in folk medicine. Among its most impressive characteristics is its effect on the female reproductive system which reacts powerfully to sage. Traditionally, sage has been used to induce late or scanty menstruation and, during menopause, normalize it. Very valuable fresh or as a dried herb, **never use sage in the form of an essential oil; the thujone content is too concentrated. Highly toxic to the central nervous system it can cause violent uterine contractions, hemorrhaging, convulsions and seizures.**

Sarsaparilla contains testosterone and progesterone; has been used to balance hormonal activity in acneic teenage young men.

The following female herbal balancers, usually used in combination are easily found prepared as extracts or in capsules.

Combo 1. *Golden Seal, Red Raspberry Leaves, Black Cohosh, Queen of the Meadow, Marshmallow Root, Blessed Thistle, Lobelia, Capsicum, Ginger, Dong Quoi.*

Combo 2. *Herbal combination for women who can't take estrogen. Golden Seal, Capsicum, False Unicorn Root, Ginger, Uva Ursi Leaves, Cramp Bark, Squaw Vine, Blessed Thistle, Red Raspberry Leaves.*

Herbal hormone balancers for both sexes include:

Combo 1. *Siberian Ginseng Root, Echinacea Root, Saw Palmetto Berries, Gotu Kola, Damiana Leaves, Sarsaparilla, Periwinkle, Garlic, Capsicum, Chickweed.*
Combo 2. *Black Cohosh, Licorice, False Unicorn, Siberian Ginseng, Sarsaparilla, Squaw Vine, Blessed Thistle.*

See also *Anti-Aging Antioxidants* and *Gourmet Ingredients* for additional hormonal oils that can be used in your everyday face recipes.

THE "R" WORD: "WRINKLES"

I'm sure you've heard the singular most important cause of wrinkling and overall skin deterioration is sun damage. Some experts believe that **90% of all wrinkles are caused by ultraviolet (UV) radiation.** Sun scorched greens are not fit for a fork, and Sun-Day Salads are definitely "out" to lunch—*anyone can prevent becoming a Sun-Day Salad.*

If, however, you are even lightly tanned, your skin has already been injured. How much damage has occurred depends on how long you have been exposed and how strong the "rays" were during exposure. Penetrating more than the epidermal shield, ultraviolet radiation causes major damage in the dermal layer. The damage is cumulative; exposure before the age of twenty can show up after 50, although changes can be seen as early as the midtwenties.

Until the 1930s, when Coco Chanel sported the first intentional tan, ladies protected their valuable complexions with parasols and bonnets. Now having discovered the damage resulting from UVs, we have come full circle and are again protecting against the searing rays with sunscreens and blocks. Totally unnecessary, wrinkles can be prevented.

SUNSCREENS

Listed as a drug, sunscreens have been hailed as, perhaps, the only "true anti-aging product in the marketplace." When used, a sunscreen not only blocks the rays, but allows your own skin's repair system to swing into high gear, reversing much of the damage, provided it hasn't progressed to precancerous or cancerous lesions. Newer sunscreens include free radical fighters and healers, vitamins A, C, E and zinc; also synthetic melanin, an oxidant that protects against both UVA (long wave, deep dermal penetrating, cumulative long-range damage) and UVB (most sunburns) radiation. Tests are being done on a vitamin C sun preparation that doesn't block the rays, but works to prevent peroxidation and cross-linking of cells, thereby avoiding UV damage.

Some cold pressed oils, especially those that are high in free radical fighting vitamins A, C and E, are mild sunscreens. See *A Splash of Oil*. Rose hip oil is especially high in vitamin C, avocado and wheat germ in E. It would make good sense to add vitamins A-C-E into these oils, for further protection. Vitamin A is available in cod liver oil, C in oil-combining ascorbyl palmitate, and oil-based E is readily found in natural and synthetic forms.

Until we have another basis for choosing a sun shield, always choose an SPF (Sun Protection Factor) 15. Which means if you begin to turn red in 5 minutes without a sunscreen and you apply an SPF 15, then $5 \times 15 = 75$ minutes (one hour and 15 minutes) is allowed before the same level of burn is sustained. You can burn while wearing a sunscreen, it just takes a little longer. When choosing a sun preparation make sure it lists SPF or "sunscreen" or "sunblock" on the label or you might be getting a tanning lotion without protection, and make sure the protection is for both UVA and UVB radiation.

Finding a sunscreen to agree with your skin can be a tricky trial and error business. Many of us have sensitivities to the ingredients in sunscreens. If you have problems with PABA, other ingredients are also efficient sunscreens. Read labels, and reread labels on products you have successfully used before, the ingredients are always changing. Depending on your skin type, choose an oil base (lasts longer, but can clog pores) or an alcohol base (drying). Unfortunately, most oil based sunscreens contain mineral oil, which will dry an already dry skin after a period of time. Look for formulas with natural oils. They cost more, but are well worth the investment.

Sensitive skins should be extra careful; many sunscreens are weak allergens. If you can't find a brand that doesn't cause itching or burning with an SPF 15, then try a lower SPF and implement with hats and protective clothing. Or, try an opaque foundation that includes chemical physical sunscreens such as titanium or zinc oxide. Some are so finely micronized that only a sheer white tonality is visible on the skin. These are also available in sunscreens.

Apply a sunscreen at least 30 minutes before being exposed to the "rays." It takes that long for the ingredients in the sunscreen to penetrate the epidermis. Apply enough, be generous. Reapply at regular intervals. If your sunscreen has an alcohol base, reapply after you come out of the water. Sunscreen all year long; UVs penetrate haze, bounce off water, snow and sand, penetrate 3 feet below water and through glass even in the car. The "rays" are stronger near the equator and on mountain tops and at higher altitudes (a tip for skiers). When applying sunscreens, always include the lips and the tops of the ears. Also, if you tan at home or in a salon, be cautious of tanning beds. Protect with both UVA and UVB blocks.

SUN-SENSITIVE

It is also important to know that some **medications, perfumes and citrus oils can increase your sensitivity to ultraviolet radiation.** Among them are hydraquinone—a skin bleaching agent; Retin-A, and excessive amounts of vitamins A and C, antibiotics, such as tetracycline, antidepressants, antihistamines, diuretics, sedatives, estrogen, birth control pills, acne medications, essential oils, germicidal soaps and antiseptics that contain hexachlorophene and bithionol, also alcohol based products, including astringents, aftershaves and colognes.

Foods that photosensitize lips to the sun are: cinnamon, celery, dill, bitter orange, parsnips, carrots, lime, bergamot (in Earl Grey tea), figs, lettuce, fennel, cucumber, corn, asparagus, mustard, onion, garlic, horseradish, artichokes, and citrus— oranges and limes (especially the juice). And you wondered why your lips became sunburned at picnics on the beach. Save the corn on the cob, sandwiches with mustard, hold the onion, dill pickles and orangeade for a picnic table under the trees. Be sure to sunscreen or block lips; they contain very little melanin.

Lighter skins are more sun-sensitive than darker skins, particularly redheads and blondes. Dark skins have the definite advantage. The darker, thicker and oilier your skin (and they go together), the less sun-sensitive you are. Darker skin has more melanin which protects against the burning rays. However, even if your skin is black, you are not protected against the more powerful rays that penetrate into the lower dermis. In short, everyone needs to protect.

SUN-DAY SOAKS: Healing Recipes

If your day in the sun, has resulted in a painful burn, before you do anything else "soak" from the inside out by **increasing your fluid intake.**

Topically pure **undiluted essential oil of Lavender is a great "soak"**—make sure it is pure and unadulterated. Almost miraculous with burns, Lavender cuts the healing time and avoids scarring.

Aloe vera is another miracle worker. Just slice open a segment and apply the gel. If no plant is available, gels and juices can be purchased in your supermarket, health food or drug store.

Strong tea (tannins) cooled, applied in compresses for 30 minutes at a time. Soaking in **baking soda** (one pound) added to a cool bath can help. Other culinary helpers are **cucumber slices topically applied, potato juice** compresses, **apple cider vinegar** compresses, **yogurt and lemon juice** and **egg white beaten together with castor oil.**

Sunburned lips can be soaked in cool compresses of **equal parts milk and water.**

SUN-DAY SUPPLEMENTS

If your body has been rapidly dehydrated from the sun, fluids and potassium need to be replaced. Free form amino acids, free radical fighters vitamins A, C, E, also zinc and bioflavonoids are all needed for tissue repair, healing and reduction of scar tissue. They are essential to destroy the free radicals released from your sunburned skin. Calcium, magnesium and B-complex are needed to reduce stress on tissues and help restore pH balance. Silicon repairs connective tissue. It may be a good idea to increase the supplements listed above before you spend time in the sun.

Note: Be cautious if taking oral PABA, a protectant for some, for others, it may cause skin problems.

THE OTHER 10%

Photoaging, as we have seen, is the major causes of wrinkles. **True aging,** if not countered, can cause some minor ones. Other causes that will immediately suggest their own solution are, **cigarette smoking, alcohol, drug and food abuse, such as yo-yo and fad dieting, missing teeth, stress and tension, lack of sleep, sleeping on your face, poor eyesight (squinting), facial grimacing and expressions, and gravity.**

A solution to gravity, that might have sounded farfetched some years ago is falling on more open minds. Yogis age very well. No doubt some of those head stands and asanas (positions) are the reason. If you can't see yourself in a head stand or similar position, the old movie stars used to swear by slant boards, not the half boards used by weight lifters, but a full body board about the length and width of a wide ironing board propped against the side of the bed. Rumors are, 5 or 10 minutes a day on a slant board and you'll never need a face lift. Slanting also helps to allign the entire body. Anyone having had a recent stroke, or who suffers from high blood pressure, or has a retinal detatchment should first see their doctor before slanting.

III.
RECIPES FOR ALL OCCASIONS

*Once thought to be a protective barrier, a one-way toxin-releasing excretory organ—it is now known that skin is a breathing, porous and permeable **two-way suit.***

"Applied to the skin, it winds up within!"

Many facial formulations do more than just lie on the surface. They can be absorbed into the lower dermal layers, your blood stream, and your internal organs—ultimately influencing overall health and function.

Whatever affects your skin, concerns your entire body, just as whatever you feed your body will absolutely show up on your skin.

*A good rule of thumb: **If you can't eat it, don't wear it!** There are few exceptions.*

THE INGREDIENTS

Open the fridge, poke around in the cabinets, it's all there right in the kitchen: water, lemon, eggs, mayo, honey, yogurt, buttermilk, heavy whipping cream, milk, tea bags, oatmeal, cornmeal, barley, wheat germ, herbs, fruits, vegetables. . . . Ingredients for good solid home cookin'—a pinch of salt, a splash of oil, a drop of vinegar, a spoonful of sugar, honey, a few basic vitamins, maybe a bottle of cod liver oil, some cooking sherry. . . . In fact, if you've been following along from the start, the only purchase you may have made is liquid protein . . . Okay, so, maybe papaya and aloe weren't on your grocery list until recently. But I'll bet you're glad they are now.

Good skin care can be had with very simple home fixings, or you may decide to become a facial gourmet. In this section, you will be offered the opportunity to be both.

RESURRECTION DRESSINGS:

TONERS

After cleansing, whether you are washing lightly, using a deep pore scrub, a "fruity peel" or an herbal facial sauna, a toner is used afterward as a second-step-cleanser to remove any residue. A toner may also be used alone, as a morning cleanser or when no makeup has been used. Creating a smooth tight protective surface, a toner will close your pores, and ideally, adjust the pH of your skin, while replacing the protective acid mantle. Some toners will invigorate, soothe and rejuvenate. With the adjustment of proportions, most of the following recipes can be adapted for dry or oily skin, and can serve as aids for blotting out blemishes and ironing out wrinkles.

DEFINITIONS

Cosmetically speaking, toners can include astringents, fresheners, pore lotions, and clarifiers. The only way to tell what you are getting is to read labels, because more often than not the terms are used interchangeably, and you may find yourself *awash* in a sea of ingredients.

Fresheners usually contain alcohol, with a smidgen of camphor or menthol—giving you a "fresh" feeling. But, then again, these are sometimes called *astringents*. The astringents or rather fresheners, or is it toners ... It's all very confusing and very drying. Just note, *any preparation that is predomi-*

101

nantly alcohol should be applied only to an oily T-zone, or Olive Oily/PotLuck Acne complexion.

Pore lotions are usually aluminum salts in a diluted low-alcohol base—just mix an antiperspirant or a teaspoon of alum in witch hazel or water that will cause your skin to swell if you want an inexpensive version of a pore lotion. Personally, I'll pass.

Clarifiers are toners that dissolve and whisk away your dead epidermal layer with the help of salicylic acid, resorcinol, benzyl peroxide and/or acetone (also used to remove nail polish). Your skin may look brighter and clearer—or redder, upset and irritated. Some "clarifiers" are very alkaline (*skin needs an acid mantle to fight off infection*), and others are extremely high in alcohol and very drying. If you are using a clarifier, I hope you don't have sensitive skin. Oh, . . . you didn't used to . . . ? Read labels and don't overdo clarifiers.

And just to add to the verbal mishmash, some astringents contain primarily citrus or witch hazel without any of the above.

"Natural" toners. Many estheticians with a natural bent, simply refer to the drying alcohol, citrus and/or witch hazel based formulations as astringent-toners and milder formulations as tonics or toners, leaving acetone and the like to the chemists. Sounds good to me. That will be our definition as well. Our astringent-toners will include pure grain alcohol or vodka, fresh fruit citrus or high quality essential oils or herbs, and ready-made witch hazel.

ALCOHOL TONERS

The use of alcohol in skin care is controversial. While alcohol can tighten pores and eliminate excess oil, it can also overtighten, strip the skin of oils, and force oil glands into high gear, creating skin that is, at once, scaly, crusty and oily. For skin that is less than oily, there is really no need for an astringent-toner on a daily basis, and for excessively oily skin, alcohol percentages in toners should not exceed 35%.

Percentages are: Normal-oily to very oily—the proportion of alcohol in your mix will vary from 5% (*1 part in 20*) or 10% (*1 part in 10*) to 35% (*about ⅓ the volume*), depending on the size of your pores and the oiliness of your skin. While normal to oily complexions can start with 5% alcohol; cut proportions if skin becomes red or irritated.

In the recipes that follow, alcohol, witch hazel and the like may be omitted and you will still have a very effective toner. The reverse is also true, should a non-astringent recipe sound good to an oily complexion, you can add astringent ingredients. Remember, your skin will dictate the proportions.

RECIPES

The following *dressings* should start your creative juices flowing and inspire culinary creativity. None of the proportions are etched in stone. *Just remember, the greater the proportions of alcohol, lemon or citrus juice, vinegar or witch hazel, the more drying the toner*. Floral waters, herbal teas, aloe juice and many fruit and vegetable juices make good non-drying toners and tonics by themselves. If mixing up a batch, all of the following must be refrigerated in clean unused bottles.

CELERY SOOTHER

Cleansing and toning, celery and rejuvenating comfrey with clarifying lemon make a "celery tonic" any Jewish deli would be proud of.

2 ounces fresh celery juice
3 ounces of strong-brewed comfrey tea (available loose or in bags in your health food store)
½ lemon

Shake the above ingredients together. Refrigerate.

"C" OR "C" COOLER

1 grated cucumber (or 1 ounce of grated celery)
1¼ cups mineral or distilled water
½ ounce tincture of Benzoin

Added options for more astringent toners:

½ lemon
5%–35% alcohol to be added to water before infusion, making
a total of 1¼ cups liquid

Place cucumber (or celery) and water in a glass bowl. Blend together with the back of a wooden spoon. Allow to infuse into the water for 1 hour. Strain out all pieces, (a coffee filter comes in handy) and you have cucumber or celery water. Add ½ ounce tincture of Benzoin. Squeeze in ½ lemon for extra toning and a little bleaching if you like. Note: if adding alcohol, be sure to add before infusing the cucumber or celery. Refrigerate.

FRUIT FANDANGOS

Fruit juices and slices make wonderful skin tonics.

Olive Oily, you may enjoy a tonic-astringent that is *half apple juice and half lemon* . . .

or, an astringent of *grapefruit juice cut with a little water and a touch of vodka.*

Lemon, grapefruit, tomato, or strawberry slices make great oily-skin "wipes."

Drier complexions can use the exfoliating enzymes in *papaya juice diluted half and half with water (a little heavier on the water) with a dash of lemon.*

Not as exfoliating as papaya, but very beneficial for **dry skin,** *peach juice may be substituted for papaya.*

In fact **Crouton Dry or Sensitives,** *just rub or pat a slice of fresh raw canteloupe, honeydew, pear, peach or apple* for a special treat.

Regular Tossed Normals can jump into the *whole fruit bowl.*

DAIRY ROYALE COMBOS

You've heard of the land of milk and honey? Peaches and cream complexions? Especially helpful for **Marinading Mature and Crouton Dry** complexions, all four ingredients are terrific toners.

Soothing on its own, **heavy whipping cream** *leaves a fatty film on the surface of the skin that helps to seal in moisture while toning.* A **slice of peach** wiped over the skin or peach juice will also soothe.

Try them together. Pulverize the pulp of a peach in a cup of heavy cream. Using the back of a wooden spoon, mash-blend the ingredients, allowing the peach to infuse into the cream for one hour. Strain out the peach bits and you have a tasty toner.

The following **wrinkle smoother** has honey for extra moisturizing: Gently warm an ounce of raw unfiltered honey in the top of a glass double boiler. When just barely warm (*don't overheat or you will destroy the enzymes and nutrients*), remove from the heat and stir in about ¾ of a cup of skim milk until the ingredients are thoroughly blended. Refrigerate. This tonic can be used twice daily.

GREAT-GRANDMA'S STAPLE!

Rosewater and Glycerine. Both Rosewater and glycerine can be **purchased at** your local pharmacy.

3 ounces of glycerine
7 ounces of triple distilled purchased Rosewater, or . . .

To make Rosewater yourself, use:

1 ounce of mashed rose buds
1 cup of water

See the preceding "C" and "C" Cooler for preparation of the "water." Or . . .

if you can afford the very expensive **essential oil of Rose,** combine:

35 drops oil of Rose
7 ounces water

Refrigerate. To add glycerine, see above for proportions.

ROSY ASTRINGENT

Proceed as above for Rosewater. Instead of using glycerine, substitute the proper proportion of alcohol needed.

ORANGE WATER AND GLYCERINE

Proceed as in *Rosewater and Glycerine* using orange flowers instead of rose buds or drops of the *essential oil of Neroli* instead of Rose.

FLORAL WATERS AND FLORAL ASTRINGENTS

All floral waters: Rosewater, Orange water, Lavender water, Chamomile, Geranium, etc., can be easily made with essential oils. *Proportions are 20 drops of oil to ½ cup of water.* See *Exotic Marinades*.

Floral preparations can be made astringent by simply adding vodka, witch hazel, essential citrus oils or juices to the recipes and cutting back on the water. For instance, an **astringent**

floral water that is excellent for acne and blemishes might include:

12 drops Bergamot (citrus)
8 drops of Lavender
4 ounces (½ cup) of water

While a **dry skin floral tonic water** could include the gentle combination of:

12 drops of either Lavender or Neroli
8 drops of Geranium or Rose; or a blend of all three
½ cup (4 ounces) of water

Be sure to refrigerate.

WITCH HAZEL WITH PIZAZZ

Used straight from the bottle, witch hazel is an old standby that has been used for centuries as an astringent. It takes on a milder character when cut half and half with a gentle soothing floral water. Or, blend the following:

THE "PIZAZZ"

1 or 2 capsules vitamin E
1 or 2 drops Chamomile oil
1 or 2 drops oil of Mint
1 or 2 drops Lemon oil
1–16 ounce bottle of Witch Hazel

HERBALESQUE

METHOD 1.

½ ounce Lavender buds
½ ounce Lemongrass
½ ounce Sweet Thyme
2 cups of distilled or mineral water
1 ounce tincture of Benzoin

Place the herbs in an enamel or heat-proof glass cookware pan with the water. When your herbal "tea" just reaches a boil, quickly reduce the heat and simmer for 5 minutes. Cool. Filter through a coffee filter or a cheese cloth. Bottle in a clean container. Add drop by drop 1 ounce tincture of Benzoin. Shake. Refrigerate.

METHOD 2.

12 drops oil of Lavender
10 drops oil of Lemongrass
8 drops oil of Sweet Thyme
6 ounces (¾ cup) water

Blend together. Do not heat. Omit tincture of Benzoin. Refrigerate. To apply, always use a cotton puff. Excellent for Oily-Acneic complexions. Avoid touching blemishes with your fingers.

VINAGRE HERBAL

Easily made, herbal vinegars balance your skin's acid mantel. They make good all over body toners and may be rubbed into the roots of your hair as well as tone the face. Astringent balancers are super for emotional oily skin flare-ups. When your skin settles down, a milder toner is in order.

Many herbalists choose a good quality white vinegar for their infusions; I prefer apple cider vinegar. *The following are diluted with floral water or a little plain distilled water before using.*

METHOD 1 (THE EASY OPTION).

20 drops of one, or a blend of several, of the following essential oils: Lavender, Rosemary, Comfrey, Chamomile, Rose, Myrtle
½ cup of vinegar

Add the essential oils to the vinegar. Blend. Before using, dilute 1:1 with distilled or spring water.

METHOD 2 (IF YOU LIKE TO PUTTER AROUND THE KITCHEN).

2 cups apple cider vinegar
1 ounce of selected flowers and/or herbs

Pour vinegar into an enamel or glass pan. Bring to just boiling. Pour over 1 ounce of dried flowers or herbs. Allow to steep for 10 days to 2 weeks, shaking daily. Before using, dilute 1:1 with distilled or spring water.

"NEW" SPICE AFTERSHAVE

For that wake up feeling, there is nothing like a good adrenal cortex stimulant. The herb rosemary is just that—stimulating and a general tonic. Proceed with either vinegar option, using the essential oil or the herb, but instead of diluting the herbal vinegar with water, use equal parts witch hazel for a tonic-astringent. Great to rub into the roots of your hair as well.

HUNGARY WATER

The following has reputed miraculous properties. According to legend, a 70 plus semi-invalid fourteenth century Hungarian Queen, stricken with gout was so restored to youth and good looks that she was courted by the King of Poland. The original recipe included cedar and turpentine, but this modern version still contains Rosemary, which is helpful in cases of gout and arthritis, and it still contains the rejuvenating oil Neroli.

4 drops of the essential oil of Rosemary
6 drops of the essential oil of Lemon
2 drops of the essential oil of Neroli
1 teaspoon triple strength Orange flower water
1 teaspoon triple strength Rosewater
2 tablespoons vodka

Blend together the essential oils. Stir the oils into the vodka. Add the floral waters. Shake thoroughly. The mixture must *mature for two months or more, but must be shaken every few days for the first couple of weeks, then once a week.* More than a toner, *Hungary Water* can be used as a light summer toilet water and mild deodorant.

ALOE TONERS

I don't think I can sing the praises of aloe too often or too loudly. There's more than a slim possibility that you could get by with aloe as the only "cosmetic" in your cupboard. Wonderful for controlling everything from acne to wrinkles, it can be used, with a little adjustment, as a toner for all skin types. And, although aloe products and straight stabilized aloe are found even in the supermarket, if you buy fresh in the produce department or grow your own aloe, you are way ahead of the game in vitality and results. A wild cactus, aloe is fairly easy to grow.

When purchasing prepared aloe, watch your *stabilizers,* ascorbic acid (vitamin C), citric acid and Irish moss are your best bets. Some of us have sensitivities to potassium sorbate, sorbic acid or other preservatives. If you've tried aloe before, and saw the reddened imprint of your hand on your itching stinging cheek for a half hour or more, it wasn't the fault of the aloe, it was the stabilizer. Read labels.

Olive Oily, Chef's T-Zone Combo, Hydrated Fruit or PotLuck Acne, opt for aloe **gel** as a toner.

Regular Tossed Normal and Chef's T-Zone Combo (on the dry side), the **juice** will do fine, or add a little vitamin E into the gel.

Marinading Mature, Crouton Dry, FridgeWorn Devitalized, **juice or gel diluted in filtered sea water** will add extra minerals from the sea.

OverSeasoned Sensitive, feel your way.

When using your own plant, scrape the gel from inside the stalk. It is easy to get the right proportions. If you are working for a *juice* consistency, moisten your skin before applying, add a very light touch of the fresh aloe gel. If you need the gel, pat it on a dry face. For extra drying, add a few drops of lemon or a little vodka; for more minerals add a little seawater; adding honey, milk, or other emollients or humectants; you can turn this mix into a moisturizer.

As you get more familiar with what your kitchen holds, you'll start to whip up your own customized versions. For instance, if your skin leans more to the oily side, you may want to try 5 parts aloe to 1 part vodka.

ALOE SURPRISE

½ cup aloe (juice or gel)
¼ cup potato or cucumber juice
½ lemon

Shake the above ingredients together. Refrigerate. The cucumber is slightly astringent and the potato will reduce puffiness. See also *Moisturizing Mists*.

EVERYDAY SAUCES:

MOISTURIZERS

Everyday sauces include **day dressings** and **nightly marinades.** They are moisturizing, lubricating and nourishing. On the whole, hardier and more "full-bodied" than toners, everyday sauces can include *olde tyme* favorites, such as whole eggs, yogurt, whipping and heavy creams, buttermilk, honey, and vegetable oils—and new time concentrates, essential oils and vitamins. The recipes can range from light oil-in-water dressings to potent intensive care marinades. Heavier dressings may be alternated with lighter ones depending on the climate in which you are living, the season, and the condition of your skin.

Every time your face and neck are cleansed, a moisturizer should be applied—gentlemen, this also includes you. Moisturizers counter water loss, keep oil and moisture balanced and protect from pore-clogging environmental dirt and make-up. Even oily skin needs a moisturizer, and dry skin should never be without. In *Spray Your Grapes and Oil Your Cucumbers,* we have seen complexions improve by misting and attracting moisture on the epidermis with humectants and hydrators. With *A Splash of Oil* water was sealed with a moisture barrier. *Everyday Sauces* will expand your menu with some delectable nutritious skin food.

DAIRY DELIGHT

1 whole egg (fertilized if you can get it)
1 tablespoon each: Plain yogurt, raw unfiltered honey (it helps to warm the spoon, to get all the honey)
⅛ teaspoon of royal jelly (the kind in a jar that needs to be kept refrigerated) (optional)
2–4 tablespoons of distilled or mineral water (more water means a lighter "delight")
4 tablespoons cold pressed vegetable oil. See A Splash of Oil *for your preference; almond, avocado and sesame are favorites.*
1 teaspoon of essential oil or blend (optional). All skin types can use Lavender, Jasmine, Neroli (orange blossom) and Rose. Or, see Gourmet Ingredients *for your skin's best choice.*

Mix all ingredients except the essential oils in a blender, then gently add the essential oils. Pour into a clean unused jar or bottle. Refrigerate and shake before using.

MARGARINE MAGIC

A wonderful moisturizer for all skin types, margarine leaves no oily residue. Found in your health food store, margarine with no artificial coloring, flavoring, preservatives, or chemicals of any kind has all the pluses for great skin care. It contains soybean oil, soy milk, vitamins A and D and skin-plumping lecithin (found in all healthy body cells). Your skin is left feeling smooth as silk.

ALOE-CREAM

A bit heavier, this little mix is dreamy-creamy, contains the vitamin "A-C-Es" and unbeatable aloe.

2 tablespoons aloe gel (fresh is best)
1 tablespoon sweet heavy cream
1 egg
3 tablespoons cold pressed veggie oil
The vitamin "ACEs" as follows:
    60,000 IU vitamin A with D (Do not use beta carotene
        unless you want a red face)
    4g–6g ascorbyl palmitate (oil-based "C"). 1g = 1000mg
    3,000 IU vitamin E
Essential oils as listed in options

Place aloe, cream, egg and oil into blender. Mix. Open capsules of ascorbyl palmitate and empty into mix. Pierce E and A caps and squeeze into mix. Blend a few seconds more. Then gently add your essential oils. Pour mix into clean bottle. Refrigerate. Shake before using.

Options: In lieu of sweet heavy cream you can try sour cream, yogurt or buttermilk. Oilier complexions may opt for more aloe gel and less oil, or choose to add a little water, possibly oil of Eucalyptus, Lemon, or Lavender. Mature or Devitalized skins need a boost in "microcirculation." This can be had with the addition of Lavender, Rosemary, Fennel and/ or Sandalwood (add individually or as a blend *10–15 drops per ounce of mix*). Try a little massage when applying. For massage, see *Wilted Salad Supreme*.

DON'T HOLD THE MAYO

One of the best moisturizer-nourishers is regular ol' mayonnaise. To ensure the highest quality, you may want to mix your own. Ingredients include protein and lecithin-rich egg yolk, extra virgin olive oil and fresh lemon juice. Can't do much better than that.

1 egg yolk
1 tablespoon fresh lemon juice
¼ teaspoon sea salt
¾ cup of extra virgin olive oil

In food processor or blender, add egg yolk, lemon juice and salt. Process 2 or 3 seconds. Then with the unit in operation, slowly and consistently drizzle the oil through the chute or top, until the "mayo" is a creamy consistency. Place in clean jar. Refrigerate.

BEFORE THE SHOWER QUICKIE

This is a personal secret. On a clean face, about 15 minutes before I take my morning shower, I squeeze a little aloe gel (about a half inch blob) into the palm of my hand, add a couple of drops of vitamin E and one drop of the essential oil of Fennel which has phytohormones similar to our own estrogen. Then I mix it around with one finger and massage it into my face and neck. If there's a little extra, it goes on whatever skin shows.

While in the humid shower, the fennel penetrates into the dermal layer along with the aloe, and the vitamin E does its work. After showering, I apply a little more cold pressed oil, usually extra virgin olive oil. Then use the ice cube method described in *Fresh From the Crisper*—giving a particular attention to the acupressure points described in the **Facelift Naturally** program. Afterward I blot, gently tapping over the points. If I need a little added moisturizing, I dab on a little extra cold pressed oil blended with the essential oils found in *Gourmet Ingredients,* or my special blend described in *Monday Marinades*. My skin feels incredible and looks it. In a few minutes, I've stimulated acupressure points, closed my pores, refined my skin with the ice, moisturized and had an aromatherapy treatment. It's a very easy, very fast and very effective routine.

EXOTIC MARINADES

Filled with gourmet ingredients, Jasmine, Angelica, Ylang-Ylang and ROSES, Geraniums, Everlast, Pine needles and Posies, this section may well be the *Nouvelle Cuisine* of skin care—*we'll have "flowers in the salad" and more flower power and exotic herbs in the marinades.* Amazing rejuvenating oils will be discovered and strange spices from ancient worlds. Reaching back into romantic biblical history, we can even opt for Frankincense and Myrrh.

The information that I will give you in this section may sound unbelievable, but without a doubt, it is real hope, not hype. The secrets of herbal healing and the epitome of natural skin care are making a resurgence today in an area called **aromatherapy.** We have touched on aromatherapy with the occasional inclusion of an essential oil, here and there, in our recipes, but now we'll get down to the nitty-gritty. All the oils we will discuss can be ordered through, or purchased at your health food stores, or mail ordered from the sources listed in *Essential Oils: Resources.*

Actually a misnomer, or a semi-misnomer, the therapy in "aroma" therapy is accomplished only in part through the "aromatic odors" of the essences. Far more interesting, the highly volatile concentrated plant oils of the herbs, roots, bark, flowers and leaves can weave their miraculous results in skin care via their ability to penetrate the epidermal and dermal layers of the skin. They rapidly find their way into the microcirculation and then travel throughout the body to encourage cell growth, and body functions via phytohormones (plant hormones), natural stimulants, balancers and soothers.

Aromatherapists have claimed major progress in areas from acne to eczema using totally natural means. I, myself, can attest to the regenerating power of essential oils for the Marinading Mature complexion.

More powerful than dried or fresh herbs, with a much longer shelf life, the concentrated aromatic oils employed by aromatherapists in skin care have also been used to help the body heal and balance itself. The penetrating oils have been employed to counter depression with essences of Clary Sage and Marjoram; blends based on Sandalwood, Jasmine, Patchouli, Clove and others. Drug addicts have been helped with Clary Sage; mental, emotional and physical exhaustion with Rosemary, Lavender and Marjoram; PMS responds to Clary Sage, Geranium, Lavender, Chamomile, Melissa, Rose and Neroli; impotency to Clary Sage, Jasmine, Rose and/or Ylang-Ylang diluted in hip baths; Pine Needle perks up exhausted masculinity; and menopause is soothed with Chamomile, Cypress, Geranium and Fennel. Stimulating essences, such as Lemon, are circulated through central air systems to help increase productivity in factories. The rarer, costly, sensual exotic essences, such as Jasmine, Neroli, Angelica and Rose, are used in only the finest perfumes. Antibacterial oils, such as Clove, Sandalwood, Basil, Rosemary, Eucalyptus, and Lavender have been known to help to hold down the "germ" count in European hospitals. Historically, the potent "aromas" have been used as protective germicides by the knowledgeable in times of plague. Not a panacea. But definitely an area to explore.

Although essential oils make you feel like royalty, I consider them basic necessities in natural skin care. Allergic reactions to essential oils are very rare, especially with external application in dilutions of 2%–3%—a definite plus. . . . Do I hear pages flipping? . . . Are you getting ready to re-read a few of those recipes that you only skimmed earlier?

Because of their price tag, many of the oils are gourmet

*fare. Some are purchased by the drop, but the highly concen-
trated essences are well worth their cost. Since the oils can
only be used by the drop, they are cost effective overall. You
will be buying quality and your skin will show it.*

In this section, you can really practice your culinary skills
with marinades, sauces and dressings that will add more punch
to your everyday "salads." **Remember in skin care, less is
more, and in aromatherapy and the use of essential oils,
this is *gospel.*** *Also be aware that some of the oils can cause
photosensitivity and should not be used directly before going
out into the sun. These oils include Rose and the citrus oils,
including Bergamot and Neroli. The essential oils will generally penetrate into the microcirculation in about twenty
minutes.*

*You will find that you will choose your personal oils by
scent. The oils that your system needs will be attractive to you.
You will also notice that many of the same oils are used for
both oily or dry complexions. There is a great deal of overlapping in functions, because many of the oils are multifunctional, working as balancing agents and oil gland
regulators. Some are rejuvenators that accelerate cell turnover
or reprogram functions; others soothe or stimulate.*

The highly concentrated volatile plant oils are listed below
according to skin type along with some traditional "starter
recipe" suggestions. The list is by no means exhaustive or
exclusive for a particular complexion, nor is your choice lim-
ited to the selection.

Regular Tossed Normal, again, has the whole Exotic Garden
to play in.

For oils listed individually, see *Gourmet Ingredients.*

MIXING THE MAGIC

To use, essential oils **must be diluted** unless otherwise
specified. Dilutions are most often made in water or cold

pressed vegetable *carrier* oils, so called because they "carry" the essence, holding it in place on the skin so that it can penetrate into the lower dermal tissue and microcirculation.

Combinations of essential and carrier oils can function as intensive care oils, rejuvenators, antiseptics, oil balancers, lymphatic stimulants, fluid and toxin drainers and more, while functioning as moisture barriers that aid in the all important oil-water balance. Essential oil can also add real zest to your ready-made creams and lotions. Dropped into distilled or spring water, the result is "scent"-sational facial tonics and toners.

Dilutions for Facial oils are usually 2½%, which measures out to be 12–15 drops of essential oil to 1 ounce of vegetable oil. But proportions can run as high as 10% for intensive treatments. A rule of thumb is to use no more than 5 or 6 different oils in one particular blend. One oil can usually do the job as well as two or more depending on the need—unless the blend is a synergy or a special combination that works more powerfully in combination and as a blend equals more than the sum of its individual parts. Synergistic blends are also included for your information.

Proportions for Floral Waters, Toners, and Tonics. Essential oils added to distilled, mineral, or spring water create **floral water toners** that can be splashed or misted on your face throughout the day. See *Resurrection Dressings* and *Moisturizing Mists.* Proportions run about 10 to 15 drops or more to 2 ounces of distilled, spring or mineral water depending on the aromatherapist, the essence used, and the purpose.

Floral waters may also be purchased as hydrosols: most delightful and soothing, hydrosols are very affordable "waters" created during essential oil distillation that contain the qualities of their more expensive concentrated oils counterparts. These may be purchased through the distributors listed in the appendix.

As with any chef, tastes differ and personal preferences exist. And, like any good chef, you will be sensitive to your own esthetic, aromatic and physical nuances, tailoring your dressings to your personal needs.

A **floral water recipe for normal to dry skin** might include *6 drops of Lavender to 4 of Rose Geranium combined in 2 ounces of water.* A **floral water for oily skin** changes the gentle Rose Geranium to a more drying citrus oil. The proportions might change, as well, to emphasize the more drying character of the floral water. *The blend would then contain 4 drops of Lavender, while the dominant citrus character of Bergamot becomes 6 drops.* A **floral water for mature skin** might combine Lavender with Frankincense or Myrrh and Neroli and/or Rose. *Or, you might try 3 drops of Geranium, 2 of Rose and 7 of Sandalwood in 2 ounces of water.* The secret is to know the properties of the oils (they are listed in *Gourmet Ingredients*) and find the scents personally attractive. The scents that attract are the ingredients your skin and body needs. The study of aromatherapy, as with culinary art, can develop into a very delicate skill that balances and blends for the occasion and need. As any great chef can attest, this is a gourmet area, indeed!

Keep floral waters refrigerated and remember to always test any new preparation on a tiny area before using. As delicious as these toners are when first mixed, they become sheer heaven after a few days of ''melding'' in the fridge.

Facial Compresses require as little as 1 or 2 drops of an undiluted essence, or premixed blend of essences, to a cup of comfortably warm water, particularly if you are using the compress to help penetrate your already applied aromatic marinades. See also *Wilted Salad Supreme* for suggestions on the facial sauna and compress.

SOAKING YOUR "HEAD!"
Traditional Marinades For Your Skin Type

Fun! Fun! Fun! Mixing, matching, marinading whether ''the head'' is a cabbage, lettuce, cauliflower, or your very own. You really can't go wrong; the rules and proportions are easy and the choices of oils are yours. Personal blends are exciting, the scents unbelievable! *By the way, aromatic oils have been used for centuries in perfumery. A drop or 2 used neat (undiluted) or blended concentrates in a little carrier oil, pure grain alcohol, or high proof vodka serve as exquisite personal signature perfumes.*

Recipes given are tried and true, while the list of *Gourmet Ingredients* will rapidly expand your culinary repertoire. Regardless of your skin type, review all recipes and experiment. You can always change the proportions or add another oil or 2. You just can't ruin your marinade. And, you might even discover that with a snappy ribbon and a pretty bottle, you've made an exquisitely personal all-occasion gift along the way.

REGULAR TOSSED NORMAL

FACE OILS

EVERYDAY

For a daily marinade, Regular Tossed, you might try scrumptious *Geranium and Lavender with exotic sensual Jasmine. Proportions 7:3:16 drops in 2 ounces of carrier oil.*

OILY ZITS DAYS

A Rosemary, Sweet Thyme, Neroli and Spike Lavender (or Lavender) blend is a **super rejuvenator** that works wonderfully for those oily zits days and is perfect for **T-Zone Combos** and **Potluck Acne!** Check *Gourmet Ingredients* and adjust the proportions for your skin type.

THE "DRYS"

A Regular Tossed having a *bout of the "drys"* might try the following intensive care moisturizing recipe:

20–30 drops Rose, Jasmine, Chamomile, Sandalwood, Lavender, and/or Frankincense in 1 ounce of carrier oil. You may want to toss in a couple of vitamin E-800s while you're mixing, also an "A" and "C" in the form of ascorbyl palmitate. If using Jasmine, go lightly; it can overpower the mix.

TONERS AND TONICS

4 drops Geranium and 7 drops Lavender in 2 ounces of water can work nicely.

But, on the whole, Regular Tossed, go for it all and have a great time!

CROUTON DRY/DEHYDRATED

Selection ideas include Geranium and Lavender to help correct endocrine imbalances associated with dry dehydrated skin. Soothing oils of choice are Chamomile, Neroli, Sandalwood and Rose.

FACIAL OILS

18 drops Geranium and 8 drops Rose in 2 ounces of carrier oil.
7 drops Geranium, 4 drops Rose, 15 drops Sandalwood in 2 ounces of carrier oil.
4 drops Rose, 6 Neroli, 12 Lavender in 2 ounces of carrier oil.

TONERS AND TONICS

10 drops Geranium and 6 drops Rose in 2 ounces of distilled water.

Also, any of the above mentioned combinations. Check *Gourmet Ingredients* for more options! Once you catch a whiff of these oils and see the results, we'll never get you out of the kitchen.

CROUTON DRY/SENSITIVE

Selection Ideas: If you are Crouton Dry and Sensitive at the same time, you will want to soothe your skin and balance your oil production. The following will help you to make your selections:

Combo #1. Very gentle soothing Chamomile, Jasmine, Neroli, Artemisia Arborescens and/or Rose.

Combo #2. Oil balancing Lavender, Geranium, and Sandalwood.

FACIAL OILS

3–4 drops Rose, 7 drops Geranium and 14 drops Sandalwood in 2 ounces of carrier oil.

10 drops Sandalwood, 4 drops Ylang-Ylang in 2 ounces of carrier oil.

TONERS AND TONICS

Any of the above oils or a blend from combos #1 and #2 added into distilled or spring water. See proportions for mixing.

OVERSEASONED SENSITIVE

Selection Ideas: Neroli, Rose, Chamomile and Artemisia Arborescens will soothe. Tread gingerly. Use a low proportion in your recipes—***no more than 10 drops essential oil*** *to 2 ounces carrier oil.* Always, test! Test! Test!

CHEF'S T-ZONE COMBO

Selection Ideas: Dear "Combo," select the oil balancers in general and, possibly, the more drying oils in the T-Zone if your condition is really extreme. Lavender, Geranium, Rosemary, Clary Sage . . . there are many possibilities. Check *Crouton Dry*, *Olive Oily* and *Gourmet Ingredients* for your personal best choice. Follow the instructions for mixing face oils and floral waters, toners and tonics at the beginning of the section.

OVERRIPE FRUIT

Selection Ideas: Geranium and Rosemary (*together stimulate lymphatic system to eliminate wastes*); Fennel (*estrogenic; do not use if epileptic*); Juniper and Lemon (*detoxify*); Patchouli (*helps eliminate excess water*).

FACIAL OIL

8 drops Geranium, 8 Rosemary, 3 Fennel, 4 Juniper, 2 Lemon, 2 Patchouli in 2 ounces of carrier oil.
Equal parts Geranium, Rosemary and Juniper (8 drops each) to 2 ounces carrier oil.

TONERS AND TONICS

Rosemary, Juniper, Lavender, Geranium and Cypress would, individually or in a blend of 2 or more, make refreshing toners and tonics. See *Mixing the Magic* for proportions.

OLIVE OILY

Selection Ideas: Geranium to balance the endocrine system; Cedarwood; astringent Cypress (or Juniper); antibacterial Sandalwood to control bacteria and reduce sebum; Bergamot to reduce oil production; Lavender to balance sebum; Rosemary to stimulate new cell formation.

FACIAL OILS

13 drops each Lavender and Bergamot in 2 ounces of carrier oil.
13 drops each Bergamot and Eucalyptus in 2 ounces of carrier oil. Also Eucalyptus and Lavender or any of the combinations above.

TONERS AND TONICS

Cypress and Juniper, together, make a **super toner.** *In 2 ounces of distilled or spring water, mix 6 drops Cypress and 10 of Juniper.*
Or, 5 drops Bergamot and 4–5 drops Lavender to 2 ounces of water.
See also Gourmet Ingredients. *There are many choices in this area:* **most important is that you like what you are smelling. This means that the oils are helping to balance your overall system. No skin condition is isolated from the entire mental, emotional, spiritual and physical you!**

ACNE

Selection Ideas: Lavender and Bergamot are both bactericidal. Lavender promotes new cell growth and is soothing, while Bergamot is astringent and antidepressant. Geranium balances the oil glands. Rosemary and Geranium stimulate the lymphatic system helping to clear toxins. Antiseptic and non-irritating Sweet Thyme (thymus vulgaris linaloliferum) is excellent for long term acne treatment. Other oils include: Myrtle, Sandalwood, Juniper.

FACIAL OILS

6 drops of Lavender, 6 of Bergamot or Neroli, 6 of Rosemary and 6 of Sweet Thyme in 2 ounces of carrier oil.
15 drops Bergamot, 11 Lavender in 2 ounces of carrier oil.
13 drops Cypress, 13 Lemon in 2 ounces of carrier oil.

TONERS AND TONICS

9–10 drops Bergamot, 6–7 drops Lavender to 2 ounces water.

ACNE ROSACEA

Selection Ideas: Bitter Orange and Mint *(to oxidize);* Linden Blossom, Rosemary and Wild Chamomile *(to detoxify).* Possibly alternated with Mint, Bay Laurel and Rosemary *(to improve facial muscles and capillary walls).* Also, Linden Blossom, Bitter Orange or Bay Laurel *(to decongest);* Lavender.

FRIDGE-WORN DEVITALIZED

Suggestion Ideas: The following synergy works very well for fatigued, sagging skin: extremely vitalizing Carrot Seed oil, Rosemary to stimulate new cell formation, Lemon Verbena for dermal waste elimination, and true Niaouli (MQV). Sandalwood is also excellent. Also, Lavender, Juniper, Hyssop, Clary Sage, Cypress.

If your skin is toxic as well as devitalized from environmental pollutants, or if you have been ill and your skin has built up toxic wastes, if you smoke or are around someone else's smoke, the following synergy will help rid your skin of the poisons and perk it up.

FACIAL OILS

9 drops each Carrot Seed oil, Rosemary, Lemongrass, and Niaouli (MQV) in 2 ounces of carrier oil.

TONERS AND TONICS

5 drops each of the same in 2 ounces of distilled water for a facial tonic.
2 drops Lemongrass, 4 Rosemary, 9 Lavender in 2 ounces of distilled or spring water.

See also Acne Rosacea *and* Gourmet Ingredients *for added ideas.*

MARINADING MATURE

Selection Ideas: Carrot Seed oil, Geranium, Neroli, Rose, Jasmine *(restore oil balance)*; Frankincense, Sandalwood, Patchouli *(counteract dullness and crepy texture)*; Fennel *(estrogen containing, wrinkle remover—**caution do not use if epileptic or on children under 6 years old**)*; Lavender *(stimulates new cell growth); Cistus* (Rock Rose) is revitalizing.

The following carrier oils are particularly good for mature skin: avocado, jojoba, peach or apricot kernel oils; also olive; or richer heavier oils, such as wheat germ, or evening primrose added into a lighter oil in a 25% dilution.

For wrinkles, especially around the eyes, try Rock Rose (rejuvenating and tightening) and Myrtle (adds elasticity, suppleness and moisture) in wheat germ oil.

FACIAL OILS

Jasmine and Rose are a great combo in an intensive treatment of 20–30 drops in 1 ounce of vegetable oil; or, cell stimulating Lavender and Neroli.

Frankincense or Myrrh (8 drops) + Lavender (13 drops) + Neroli (3 drops) in 2 ounces of vegetable oil. Play with proportions, add in lecithin caps, vitamins A, C, E. See Monday Marinades *for mixing in thick lecithin and vitamins.*

TONICS AND TONERS

Any of the above oils either separately or blended. See *Mixing the Magic* for proportions.

REJUVENATING SKIN OILS

Geranium, Frankincense, Jasmine, Lavender, Neroli *(all hormonal)*, Rosemary *(stimulates new cell formation)*; Carrot Seed *(vitalizing)*; Myrtle for suppleness, elasticity, moisture; Rock Rose (cistus) rejuvenating and tightening; Everlast *(stimulation of new cell growth)*; also Clary Sage and Rock Rose *(fine lines)*, Chamomile, Patchouli, Rose.

All of the preceding information includes recipes and oils that have been used traditionally by aromatherapists and can serve as points of reference. Warm compresses can be used over the facial oils to aid in penetration. 1, 2 or 3 drops of the above oils may be added into the compresses, as well.

The essential oil distributors listed in the appendix, among others, are sincerely working to bring you the highest quality oils and products, and are conscientiously researching in a field that has already been established as accepted healing for more than thirty years in Europe. If you are interested in this area of self skin care, write for their catalogs and price lists. Most have ready mixed preparations as well as oils for personal formulations. Books and courses are also available.

For more information on the more commonly used oils, see *Gourmet Ingredients*.

GOURMET INGREDIENTS
(HERBS AND ESSENTIAL OILS)

A wealth of regenerative healing power for your fabulishous face is quick referenced below. Be advised that herbs and plants in the form of concentrated essential oils **must be diluted** in your recipes. Cold pressed vegetable oil, alcohol, vinegar, or water are used or the essences can be mixed directly into prepared beauty creams. Never use an essential oil neat (undiluted) unless specifically indicated.

Reviewing the list, you will find that many of the oils are used for conditions that seem totally incongruous. Multifunctional, aromatics can work to balance extreme conditions and on many levels, from the physical to the mental-emotional. For instance, Lavender balances sebum production, so it can be used for the extremes of acne, as well as dry skin and it is also sedating.

When you select your gourmet ingredients, consider the healing and regenerative qualities they hold on the physical level, but choose those aromas that most attract you. You will automatically gravitate to the oils you need. They will please, relax and pamper.

Advantages of this gourmet fare include penetration beneath the outer skin to rejuvenate subcutaneous dermal tissue. Preparation requires no boiling, steeping, or waiting. Application is simple. And the normally long shelf life of essential oils can be further extended when kept in a cool dark place or refrigerated.

Listed are some of the most commonly used oils in skin care, a few of the rarer ones, and some general rules for preparation.

Artemisia Arborescens. Anti-inflammatory and strengthening; very important in skin care. Particularly beneficial for extremely OverSeasoned Sensitive, it may be used for all skin types.

Anti-inflammatory, non-irritating oils. German Chamomile, Everlast, Artemisia Arborescens, Rose. (Anti-inflammatory oils that can be slightly irritating include Lavender, Eucalyptus Citriodora, Melissa.) Used to soothe and quiet all skins.

Astringent oils. Cypress, Geranium, Cedarwood, Frankincense, Juniper, Myrrh, Patchouli, Peppermint, Rose, Rosemary, Sandalwood, Lemon, Tangerine.

Bath. Dilution: about six drops sprinkled over the water and well-mixed with your hand before entering. The highly volatile oils dissipate rapidly so enter the bath immediately. OverSeasoned Sensitive skins, add your essential oils to a little whole milk, a carrier oil or egg yolk before adding it to the water. Most all gourmet ingredients listed may be used for bathing. **Note:** These recipes are not meant for babies or young children.

Benzoin. Strange spicy heady incensy benzoin is actually a resin not an oil, but a gourmet ingredient nonetheless. Benzoin relieves irritation, itching, cracking and redness. With Lemon or Lavender it makes a lovely hand cream; also, Benzoin is a good fixative that stabilizes blended "recipes." When purchasing, make sure this thick resinous ingredient has been diluted in wood alcohol rather than ethyl glycol. If not diluted, you will have to heat benzoin over a pot of boiling water to dissolve and use it.

Bergamot. Citrus scented antiseptic Bergamot is a preferred oil in acne/oily skin care recipes. It is also very effective for herpes, skin ulcers and wounds, fighting staph and various other forms of bacteria. Used in compresses, in toners and skin moisturizing oils, its citrus scent is appreciated by both men and women. Mixed with Eucalyptus, another potent anti-viral oil, Bergamot can be used neat or mixed with a little alcohol and dabbed on the individual herpes simplex eruptions. *Note: Never use undiluted as an all over face or body oil, or when going out into the sun. All citrus oils photosensitize the skin for several days after application. Burning can result, particularly if undiluted.*

Camphor. Useful for Olive Oily and PotLuck Acne complexions, also helpful applied neat with a cotton swab for pimples and warts. Otherwise, *other oils* are more useful in general skin care recipes.

Carrier oil. A carrier can be almost any unscented vegetable oil used to dilute concentrated "gourmet" essences. Their main purpose is to lubricate and hold the aromatic oils on the skin allowing the more concentrated oils to be absorbed into the dermal tissue and system. Some have therapeutic value as well. See *A Splash of Oil.*

Carrot (Daucus Carota). A must for FridgeWorn Devitalized or Marinading Mature complexions, Carrot is a very effective revitalizer. Traditionally used to treat skin ulcers and even skin cancers, Carrot Root contains beta carotene, Vitamins B1, B2 and C. Wonderful for all skin types, Carrot can restore tone and elasticity as well as reduce wrinkling. Smells just like a carrot.

Cedarwood. A selected ingredient for mild astringent recipes, Cedarwood is a powerful antiseptic that is valuable for Potluck Acne and Olive Oily complexions. Gentlemen, you will love the masculine scent. Also a selection for alopecia (baldness), dandruff and seborrhea of the scalp. Ladies, do not use if pregnant.

Celery (Appium Graveolens). Particularly effective for eczema.

Chamomile (Blue, German). A most effective anti-inflammatory ingredient with an apple-like scent, Chamomiles come in several different varieties. For our recipes we are looking for either the Roman (Anthemis Nobilis) or the German (Matricaria Chamomila) types. Azulene-containing Chamomile cools, soothes and is non-irritating. A vasoconstrictor causing small blood vessels to shrink, Chamomile reduces redness in the cheeks. This gourmet ingredient can be very useful in preparations for acne rosacea although it may take months for noticeable improvement. Note: Sometimes with natural healing herbs and oils, there is what is called a ''healing crisis'' where the condition sometimes appears to worsen before improvement is seen. The Chamomiles are so gentle, however, that Chamomile is one of the few oils that have been used traditionally in the treatment of children. Very effective in extremely low dilutions, Chamomile is wonderful for all skin types from PotLuck Acne, to Crouton Dry, to OverSeasoned Sensitive to Marinading Mature, soothing irritation and burns as well. A breathtakingly yummy scent, especially fresh from the fridge mixed in cold, cold water as a facial splash. Wonderful in combination with Lavender.

Clary Sage. This gourmet ingredient has a sweet nutty aroma producing a euphoric effect on those using it, but can cause nightmares if used when drinking alcohol. Utterly warming and relaxing, if applying Clary as an overall body oil or for massage, do not drive afterward; you might fall asleep. Used with benefit by all complexions from Regular Tossed Normal to OverRipe Fruit, anti-inflammatory and tonic Clary Sage cools inflamed skin. For very oily hair and dandruff, a couple of drops in the rinse water produces positive results.

Compress. To prepare a compress with essential oils, dilute 2–4 drops in a bowl of warm or cool water. See *Wilted Salad Supreme*.

Cypress smells exactly like the tree. Cypress is styptic (*stops bleeding*) and is very astringent. A vasoconstrictor, it is excellent for ''broken capillaries,'' which are really not broken at all, but stretched out. If used twice a day for months, results may be seen. Effective in recipes for Olive Oilys and OverHydrated Fruits, Cypress will help to balance both.

Evening Primrose Oil. Definitely a gourmet ingredient, but not an essential oil, a capsule of Evening Primrose can add value to your carrier oils. Found in your health food store in the vitamin area, Evening Primrose Oil, contains GLA (gamma Linolenic acid) used by the body to make hormone-like substances called prostaglandins. See *A Splash of Oil* and *Plant Food Plus*.

Eucalyptus. Eucalyptus comes in a whopping 300 or more varieties. All have very powerful bactericide with anti-viral properties—the chemical reaction of Eucalyptus produces ozone in the air, an environment in which bacteria cannot live. Although Eucalyptus Globulus is most often found, the gourmet's gourmet might choose calming lemony **Eucalyptus Citriodora** or **Eucalyptus Dives** for skin care. Effective on septic or congested skin, Eucalyptus limits excess sebum production in PotLuck Acne and Olive Oily complexions and is often applied neat with a cotton swab on pimples. A water balancer for Overhydrated Fruit complexions, Eucalyptus is also a tissue regenerator with mild estrogenic properties. It is helpful in burn healing, particularly in combination with Lavender and is useful in compresses for post operative dressings. Applied neat on herpes simplex I (cold sores), blisters and shingles, it can also relieve chicken pox. See also *Bergamot*.

Everlast (AKA Strawflower, Helichrysum Ital. Serot.). Important for new cell formation, Everlast is the strongest natural anti-inflammatory in the essential oil repertoire. It prevents bruising and counteracts swelling.

Face oils. Essential oil dilutions for face recipes are usually 2½–5%, sometimes running as high as 10% for intensive treatments. A 2½% dilution is about *15 drops essential oil to 1 ounce of carrier*. You will be using a dropper to measure out your oils and may also be using a bottle from the drug store. *A 30 ml bottle contains 1 ounce*.

Fennel. Estrogenic Fennel is an anti-wrinkle oil that can balance OverHydrated Fruit complexions. *Caution: Do not use on children. Avoid if epileptic*.

Frankincense (AKA Olibanum). A heavy penetrating camphoresque essence of exotica, Frankincense is a must for Marinading Mature skin, It adds tone, erases wrinkles and preserves a youthful complexion, rejuvenating by speeding up growth cells.

Ginseng. Though not an essential oil, Ginseng is definitely gourmet fare and is often used in conjunction with aromatherapy for its tonic and stimulating effects. A welcome addition to masks and facial saunas, Ginseng Root is an excellent skin conditioner and cleanser.

Geranium (Perlargonium Odorantissimum; also, Perlar Capitatum—Rose Geranium). A very flowery ''green'' scent that an untrained nose might mistake for Rose, particularly the variety known as ''Rose'' Geranium which is sometimes used to adulterate or extend the more expensive Rose oil. Altogether refreshing, Geranium is a balancer that can work for all complexions from OverRipe Fruit to sluggish congested Olive Oily to Crouton Dry. Cleansing and refreshing, it is one of the few oils whose fresh fragrance can blend with any oil. Strongly astringent, this lymphatic stimulator releases fluid from watery complexions, yet is soothing to dry irritated skin. Antiseptic and mildly analgesic and sedative, this mild skin tonic comforts neuralgia pain, heals burns and ulcers and comforts inflamed skin. Note: if you have highly sensitive skin, eczema or dermatitis, this *may not* be the oil for you.

Hormonal oils. Some of the more popular essences containing phytohormones that imitate estrogen are Cypress, Clary Sage, Savory, Parsley, Thyme, Angelica, Cajeput, Geranium, Fennel, Hops, Chamomile and Eucalyptus (slightly).

Inula graveolens. Loosens pore-clogging sebum, excellent for Olive Oily and congested overactive complexions.

Jasmine. A very expensive, heady, long-lasting, erotic, animal-like sweet scent that can be used by all skin types. Crouton Dry and Sensitive, in particular, love recipes that include Jasmine. Jasmine counters itching and redness and can calm dermatitis especially when accompanied by *depression*. One of the more costly oils, a very little goes a long long way.

Juniper. A detoxifier, an antiseptic and a diuretic that reduces excess water in the skin, Juniper is an excellent choice for Olive Oily, OverHydrated Fruit and PotLuck Acne. Diluted in spring or mineral water, Juniper makes an astringent skin tonic or toner with a pleasant masculine woodsy odor.

Lavender. Barring Aloe and Tea Tree oil, Lavender is the closest ingredient to a skin care panacea in the entire niche of gourmet treasures. Undoubtedly the most used and versatile of all the oils, calming, soothing and balancing Lavender, applied neat to burns, is said to increase the rate of healing. It is a most potent stimulator of healthy new skin cells, healing wounds quickly. Highly valued by PotLuck Acne complexions, Lavender (and Spike Lavender), often combined with Bergamot, can reprogram acne/oily skin. Sebum production is balanced, scarring reduced, bacterial growth is inhibited, while the skin is soothed. Along with Neroli, Lavender rejuvenates Marinading Mature skin and may be chosen to help in cases of eczema. Both the herb and the essential oil are used in everything from washes to toners, moisturizers and masks. Although slightly irritating to the most highly sensitive complexions, Lavender is a "can't go wrong" choice for most all complexions.

Lemon (Citrus Limonum)—A powerful bactericide, Lemon is also used as a mild skin bleach to lighten and brighten discolored areas, particularly on the neck. A powerful degreaser that is helpful in treating Olive Oily and greasy skin, Lemon has been used highly diluted to mend "broken capillaries." See also *Cypress*. Easily irritating, especially to sensitive skin, 2 drops of Lemon is enough in a bath, and cut back to 1% dilutions in your mixed oils as well.

Lemongrass. Antibacterial against staph, antiseptic, a good skin tonic, Lemongrass spells acne control, it is a cleanser for oily skin. As with Lemon, use in low dilutions.

Melissa (Lemon Balm). Very rare and expensive, true Melissa soothes the body and the mind. Although most often used to treat skin conditions like eczema or allergies, take care to use Melissa in dilutions of only 1% or you could intensify the very condition you are trying to alleviate. This means that if you use the oil in a bath, use no more than a safe 3 or 4 drops to a full tub. Often Melissa will seem to intensify a condition briefly, but a part of the healing process, this will subside. Most often, when purchased it is cut with oil of Lemongrass, Lemon or Verbena. Melissa is usually used if Chamomile hasn't helped.

Myrrh. A pungent spicy resin known for its use in incense, Myrrh is filled with biblical romance and exotic undertones. Anti-inflammatory, it can also rejuvenate Marinading Mature.

Myrtle. Astringent, antiseptic and bactericidal properties make Myrtle a good choice in PotLuck Acne and Olive Oily recipes.

Neroli (Orange Blossom or Citrus Auranthium). Possessing the exquisitely soothing scent of an orange blossom, this is an oil around which legends of romance have been built. A hormonal oil, Neroli acts at the cellular level, regenerating tissue, preserving the health and youth of all complexions, especially Marinading Mature. Non-irritating, Neroli functions well even if your complexion is red or irritated. It is an excellent choice for dry, broken skin with noticeable capillaries.

Niaouli (True; MQV). A powerful tissue stimulator. With properties ranging from anti-allergic to antiseptic, this oil is very versatile. It has been a recommended choice in combination with Carrot Seed oil, Rosemary and Lemongrass to stimulate FridgeWorn Devitalized complexions, strengthening the skin's metabolism.

Palma Rosa. An antiseptic cellular stimulator, this scented grass offers an essential oil that smells somewhere between roses and geraniums. A valuable skin care oil, it hydrates Crouton Dry, and perks up Marinading Mature. Like Lavender and Neroli, and several others, Palma Rosa stimulates cellular regeneration, while calming OverSeasoned Sensitive and inflamed skin.

Patchouli. Patchouli has a very strange almost animal scent—musty, heavy and lingering—sometimes for weeks. Some say it smells like old attics and worse, but it is nonetheless a valuable aid in skin care. Anti-inflammatory and antiseptic, Patchouli is also a water balancer and skin rejuvenator that calms red skin, dries weeping sores, and, at the same time, heals cracked skin. It is very helpful in some forms of eczema, fungal infections and skin allergies. Most helpful to PotLuck Acne complexions.

Peppermint. A relief for most any kind of skin itching and irritation, including sunburn, Peppermint must be used in low very dilutions (under 1%); higher can cause aggravation of the condition. Antiseptic, Peppermint combines for a refreshing toner that can also be used to soothe inflammation and redness. PotLuck Acne, especially, might find soothing comfort here in the form of a toner, and relief for skin congestion with a facial steaming. Good for all skin types in very low dilutions.

Rock Rose (Cistus Ladaniferus). Rejuvenating and tightening. Combined with the essential oils of Rose and Myrtle, Cistus is often used to soften fine lines in the eye area.

Rose. Very costly, the price soars over $1000.00 an ounce (of course you may not wish to buy a full ounce). Still, the effects of this four star gourmet ingredient is affordable as a soothing hydrosol, an aromatic water that is a by-product of the essential oil processing. An excellent toner for dry skin, Rose hydrosol can be purchased at a comfortable price, and the effects of this soothing antiseptic skin tonic can be had by all. Rose is particularly loved by Marinading Mature skin, Crouton Dry and OverSeasoned Sensitive, offering a delicious psychological lift as well. Very beneficial for faces with thread veins on the cheeks. It is anti-inflammatory and astringent, Rose tones the capillaries just below the skin, although real improvement may not be seen for weeks.

Rosemary. Rosemary is a tradition in skin and hair care. Reputed by Queen Elizabeth of Hungary to bestow miraculous benefits in the legendary "Hungary Water," it is a cell regenerator, stimulating new cell formation, while balancing excess fluid in the skin. Generally used as a tonic-astringent in skin care, this stimulating and cleansing herb is also used as an "after the shampoo" rinse for dark hair, and has helped cases of dandruff and baldness.

Rosewood. A floral-woody-spicy scent marks this delightful oil. A gentle emollient, Rosewood, at once, calms and stimulates skin cells. Wonderful, especially for Crouton Dry and Sensitive skin.

Sage. Definitely a gourmet ingredient well known for its place in the culinary arts, Sage balances excess fluid. It is tonic, good for sluggish or congested skin and is a skin regenerator. An herb to be respected, Sage is to be used as a **dried herb only.** Although an excellent skin regenerator, the essential oil can be toxic even in the smallest doses, possibly inducing uterine spasm and convulsions. Ladies, **do not use when pregnant.** For an herb that functions like Sage, minus the toxic effects see *Clary Sage.*

Sandalwood. A powerful antibacterial against staph and strep and a mild astringent, Sandalwood is an excellent choice for PotLuck Acne. Wonderful for Crouton Dry and Dehydrated complexions, warm compresses of Sandalwood relieve itching and inflammation.

Skin tonics. Bergamot, Geranium, Camphor, Cypress, Juniper, Peppermint, Rose (the only toner recommended for dry skin), Rosemary, Lemongrass and Clary Sage.

Spearmint. The dried herb in facial steam cleanses and refines pores.

Tangerine. Super astringent for oily skin

Tea tree (Melaleuca Alternifolia). An essential oil that has many uses. A medicine chest in a bottle, Tea Tree is an immune stimulant, a wound healer that becomes more potent in the presence of infection. Used full strength and dabbed on the "spots," Tea Tree is very helpful for PotLuck Acne complexions. Antiseptic, it soothes irritated skin. It is also antibacterial, a fungicide, topically used on pimples, boils, burns, sunburn, stings, cuts, splinters and ringworm. Non-toxic Tea Tree preserves healthy tissue and promotes healing, while diminishing the possibility of scarring. It is an oil that should be in every home.

Thyme, Sweet (Thymus Vulgaris Linalol). *(Pronounced time)* A special non-toxic non-irritating chemotype, this is the only Thyme that is safe for home use as an essential oil. Controlling micro-organisms, it is an excellent choice for long term treatment of acne. Sweet Thyme is also used in the treatment of hair loss.

Ylang-Ylang. (Pronounced *ee-lang ee-lang*) This heavy, heady, sweet oil, traditionally used as an aphrodisiac, can be balanced by blending with a citrus note like Bergamot or Lemon. Ylang-Ylang balances sebum production, soothing Olive Oily to Crouton Dry skin. Use in low doses to avoid a possible headache. Some skin sensitization in a small percentage of people has resulted from the use of this oil.

MASQUES DE MAISON & MASQUES EXOTIQUES

A masque, or mask (sounds the same and is the same) may be nothing more than a squashed banana, pressed grapes, or a cooked carrot mashed with a little honey; you'll find these under *Masque de Maison*. A mask can also be a highly targeted herbal or aromatic oil-laced preparation that addresses specific problems, this is a *Masque Exotique*

MASQUES DE MAISON

"De Maison," French for *of the house,* the *masques* in this section include ingredients that are for the most part kitchen available. Readily found *around the house,* they are masques that you can put together without going through any extra shopping.

A *masque de maison* can be a simple coating of plain yogurt, honey or egg white, a glob of precooked oatmeal or oat flakes soaked in water, yogurt, witch hazel, buttermilk, fruit, vegetable or aloe juice. In fact, cooked or uncooked, oatmeal makes a fantastic mask that soothes sensitive skin, calms irritations, draws excess oil out of oily skin and cleanses beautifully. You can also opt for a lush peaches and cream complexion—peaches and heavy cream, that is . . . or, strawberries and whipping cream. Yummy!

Once you get the idea that you are actually allowed to just "hang out" with "egg on your face" and can luxuriate in the

notion that a napkin or towel exists only to catch trickles of
sweet scented fruit juices or dollops of warm gooey oatmeal,
mashed carrots or potato as you hedonistically lay relaxing on
your bed swathed in your favorite food or, better yet, soaking
in an aromatic bath, you will be well on your way to fabu-
lishously succulent skin.

Usually associated with an elaborate facial, as in *The Wilted
Salad Supreme,* masks can also be applied without intense
preparation. There is really only one rule for masks—*place
them on clean faces.* Your mask will deep clean, tighten and
feed your skin, help to unclog pores, increase the circulation,
and cell turnover. And, depending on the ingredients, it can
also reprogram dermal tissue and resurrect aging skin with the
use of aromatic herbs and essences as in *Masques Exotiques.*

Fruits, vegetables, dairy products and oatmeal, clays, yeasts
and sweets provide the basis for a *Masque de Maison.*

BASICS TO BUILD ON

CHOOSING YOUR INGREDIENTS

The ingredients you choose will depend on your skin type,
the attention it needs and the food in the fridge. This chapter
will give you a free hand to experiment with your ingredients.
You really can't go wrong. All you need is enough "stuff"
to adequately cover your face. Stuff that won't dry and crack
in 15–20 minutes. The following hints may be used as guides.

Oatmeal soothes.
Yeast stimulates.
Vegetable oils add emollients
Honey and egg hydrate.
Lemon cuts through oil and bleaches; all *citrus* astringes.
Fruits, especially papaya, pineapple, grapes exfoliate, also *but-
     termilk.* (Most all of the ingredients listed exfoliate to
     some degree.)
Egg tightens.

To expand your list See *Skin Juices.*

SWEET TIMES

Marinading Mature, Crouton Dry and OverSeasoned Sensitive skins eat up this recipe.

2 teaspoons honey
5 drops hazelnut and or rose hip seed oil

To make this a masque "exotique" simply add 1 or 2 drops of an essential oil or blend according to your skin type. See *Masques Exotique* and *Gourmet Ingredients.*

Optional ingredients:
Crouton Dry, PotLuck Acne: *add egg yolk.*
Olive Oily skin: *add egg white.*
Sensitive: *add 1 or 2 drops of Celery Seed oil.*
To lighten brown spots: *add lemon juice (or essential oil) or essential oil of Fennel, also Aloe.*
For added stimulation: *a dash of brewer's yeast.*
For added minerals, *chlorophyll or a capsule of spirulina.*

YEAST CAKES

Nutritional or brewer's yeast is a very effective foundation for a tightening and stimulating mask, although it is sometimes irritating to OverSeasoned Sensitive skin. Crouton Drys and Marinating Matures might want to "oil up" a little before applying a mask that is primarily made with yeast, or rather use yeast as a minor ingredient in a fruit or veggie combo. For a super recipe see *Specialties of the House: Skin Tighteners, The Youthful Yeast Yummy.* Nutritional yeast may also be added to oatmeal, yogurt-oatmeal, honey and egg recipes.

MAKING MUD PIES: CLAYS

What? You say, you don't eat clay? You thought we washed this off of the salad? Well, just in case you weren't aware, some clays are edible and come in capsules for internal cleansing and use as mineral supplements.

TYPES OF CLAYS

Deep-cleansing, toxin-absorbing clays can be distinguished by color and may be purchased in your health food store:

Green clay reduces oil production and is used for Olive Oily skin. It has a high concentration of chromium, nickel and copper.

White clay is milder than green. It is almost pure aluminum oxide with small quantities of zinc oxide and works very well to balance oil production and detoxify a Chef's T-Zone Combo or a Regular Tossed Normal with a moderately oily T-Zone.

Blue clay, anti-inflammatory, is excellent for OverSeasoned Sensitive or PotLuck Acne. The blue color comes from the cobalt salts it contains.

Red clay, high in iron, works well for Regular Tossed Normal skin.

Pascalite clay contains many minerals, including aluminum, barium, boron, cadmium, calcium, chromium, cobalt, copper, gallium, iron, magnesium, manganese, nickel, potassium, silica, sodium, strontium, titanium, vanadium, and zirconium. It is the clay that is generally rated as safe (GRAS) by the FDA for internal use as a mineral supplement and can be used for all skin types.

MIXING IT UP

2 tablespoons of clay according to skin type

Enough distilled or spring water and/or juice (water and aloe make a good combo), or herbal teas to make a great slippery mud pie.

1 teaspoon hazelnut and/or rosehip seed oil (in a pinch use any good cold pressed oil)

Optional: A few drops of vitamins E and A or a little cod liver oil.

First **mix** the clay and liquid. Then add your oils and other ingredients. When **applying** a clay mask, always apply it in at least a ⅛ inch thick layer, and leave it on for no more than 15 minutes. A thin clay mask will dry too quickly and dehydrate even the most OverRipe Fruit complexion. Never allow a clay mask to dry totally. The drier and more delicate your complexion the shorter the time of application. When you use a clay mask avoid your sensitive eye area. Place cool compresses over your eyes while relaxing. See recipes in *Buffet Style Eye-Sings*.

MASQUE-R"ADES"

SKIN TYPES AND BEST BETS

Chef's T-Zone Combos do best if clay is applied to only the oily areas.

OverSeasoned Sensitive does best with honey and yogurt, some melon and grape. Honey mixed with finely ground almonds or oatmeal makes a good non-irritating mask. Also pulverized cucumber and yogurt.

Very Olive Oily, PotLuck Acne and **OverRipe Fruit** benefit greatly by the application of a clay mask. It will draw out impurities and toxins, while tightening and minimizing pores. A dash of brewer's yeast adds to the extractive quality, while adding "B" vitamins. Cabbage juice, grape and tomato juice and pulp can be added singularly or in pairs to the clay for PotLuck Acne Complexions. Olive Oily skin can benefit from the same, with the additional selection of pear, lemon, or strawberry.

Regular Tossed Normals should use a clay mask no more than once a month and fruit masks arc not really needed more than once a week. All fruits and oils can be used by Regular

Tossed Normals from astringent lemons, grapes and peaches to the rich avocado and wheat germ oils. And if the fruits are runny, a tablespoon of clay, or oatmeal can be added for body.

Crouton Dry, Fridge-Worn Devitalized and Marinading Mature complexions should generally elect to use a clay-free, or almost clay-free recipe, since clay can absorb 200 times its weight in water and can be very dehydrating. A mashed avocado makes an excellent mask for **Crouton Dry** and **Marinading Mature** skin, as do carrots, bananas and melons with the addition of nutritious, moisturizing wheat germ oil which is high in vitamin E. The mildness of fruit or mashed cooked carrot is ideal with a little honey for moisture. Honey may even be used alone, or mixed with mashed avocado pulp or banana. Ground almonds mixed with a little honey also make a good mask for mature skin.

SPECIAL AREAS THAT BENEFIT FROM "MASQUES"

The infamous **T-Zones.** Here clays can blot up excess oil, toxins and clean the pores.

"Fine line" areas like "crowsfeet," "parentheses" at sides of mouth and upper lip "puckers" found in Crouton Dry and Marinading Mature skin need the dead skin lifted away and circulation stimulated. Green papaya is good mixed with a little clay, oatmeal or brewer's yeast—just be sure to moisturize immediately after rinsing off your mask.

Olive Oily and **PotLuck Acne** skin can use clay masqus more than most to help balance oil production.

OverRipe Hydrated and **FridgeWorn Devitalized** need feeding masks that may include yeast. It will activate circulation, bringing blood, oxygen and nutrition to the face. See *The Youthful Yeast Yummy*.

MASQUES EXOTIQUES

With the addition of essential oils to your *Masques de Maison,* they become *"Masques Exotique."* As in the *Exotic Marinades,* some of the essential oils mentioned here are very *exotique* indeed, and can be purchased only from a very few suppliers, while others are more easily found.

One to four drops of these very concentrated oils are used per mask depending on the thickness and the total volume of ingredients used. If you use more than a single oil, be sure to mix up your blend or blends in advance.

OverRipe Fruit. Lavender and/or Juniper into clay.

Regular Tossed Normal. Neroli (Orange Blossom), Jasmine, Lavender.

Crouton Dry, Marinading Mature. Sandalwood (for *dryness*), Fennel *(estrogenic wrinkle eraser, do not use if epileptic),* Carrot Seed Oil *(restores tone and elasticity),* Frankincense *(speeds up cell growth),* Patchouli, Neroli (Orange Blossom), Myrrh, Lavender *(very cytophylactic, stimulating growth of new cells),* gentle Rose, Rock Rose, Myrtle, or Rose Geranium *(contains phytohormones).*

OverSeasoned Sensitive. Roman Chamomile, Lavender, Everlast (Strawflower), Great Mugwort (Artemisia Arborescens) (soothing *and anti-inflammatory).* These oils work together synergistically. They function to soothe the skin, calm inflamed blood vessels, counter inflammation, muscular spasms, swelling and bruising, easing physical, as well as, emotional tensions, while stimulating new cell formation. The gentle essential oils of Neroli (Orange Blossom), and Rose also soothe.

Potluck Acne *(Also of great benefit to Regular Tossed Normal).* Spike Lavender, Neroli, Rosemary, Thyme. A synergistic group, these oils function in several ways; they are nonirritant, antiseptic; stimulating new cell formation, metabolism, circulation and toxin removal in the dermal layer. The blend contains plant hormones to regenerate tissue, while re-programming dermal tissue gently and safely.

Acne rosacea. Blue (German) Chamomile. See also *Acne rosacea.*

Dry skin acne. Lavender (Lavendula Vera), Spike Lavender, Clary Sage, Geranium (Pelargonium Asperum), Petigrain.

PotLuck Acne, overactive, oily. (Do not use if using cortisone). A synergistic combination of Spike lavender, Rosemary, Inula Graveolens, Eucalyptus encourages new cell growth, oil glands rebalance, pores are unclogged, and dermal tissue is re-programmed, while leaving the protective oil layer intact. Also of value—Frankincense.

FridgeWorn Devitalized, Crouton Dry, stressed out skin, or basically healthy skin that is tired and saggy. Helpful if exposed to heavy environmental pollution; helps detoxify smoker's skin. Lemongrass, Carrot Seed oil, true Niaouli (MQV), and Rosemary. An intensely revitalizing combo stimulates new cells, while coaxing dermal tissue to release toxins; also, Eucalyptus Globulus, Myrtle and Neroli.

IN GENERAL ...

The preceding suggestions will give you an idea of what can work for whom. A mask needs no more than one or two fruits and/or one or two essences. The same aromatic ingredients you use in your toners and moisturizers can be used in your masks, only the overall proportions change.

For most skins, cleansing masks may be used weekly, oily T-zones twice weekly. Regular Tossed Normal can do with "treatment" masques every now and then, while Over-Seasoned Sensitives should avoid heavy "treatment," using only the more gentle, fruits, vegetables, honey, and oat or almond meals.

All masks (including fruits, honey, etc.) are left on for up to twenty minutes (clay masks for less) then, gently softened with warm water, or a cloth soaked in warm water and thoroughly rinsed. Splash about 20 to 30 times, then blot dry.

Regular use of these masks will provide lasting rejuvenating results, especially with the addition of essential oils. However, if you feel you can't spend the t-i-m-e to fit in the relaxing fifteen or twenty minutes once a week it generally takes for a mask to work its magic (. . . although once you've tried it and seen the results . . .) a nightly *masque de maison* "quicky" can include a simple layer of aloe gel followed by a layer of plain yogurt. Both can be rinsed off in the morning. After a few nights, you'll be surprised at the difference in the texture and tone of your skin. A little pulverized cucumber mixed with yogurt will calm and soothe even the most sensitive skin. This, too, can be used daily by all skin types.

Additional recipes and/or ingredients may also be found under the individual skin types section. See also *Scrub Those Carrots* . . . for exfoliating masks and *Gourmet Ingredients* to expand your repertoire.

MONDAY MARINADES:
INTENSIVE TREATMENTS

It's Monday and you're feeling blue, a little tired . . . dried out . . . and your skin shows it. You're taking the day off, kicking back, shelving all work, playing hooky . . . You've captured "the Monday Marinade moment." Marinading Mature, Crouton Dry, FridgeWorn, *Monday Marinades* are yours for life. Used all week long, they will become your Sunday Soaks, Tuesday Tonics, Wednesday Wonders, Thursday Thirst Quenchers, Friday Frolics and well, you've got the idea.

If this is the first time you are using an intensive treatment, you will find your face soaks it up instantly. Your skin may even ask to be fed twice a day. Fabulous for application after a facial or mask, most all complexions can benefit, Olive Oily as well; just blot off the excess after a 20 or 30 minute treatment.

Free-radical fighters, vitamins A-C-E, the battling *"Aces,"* nutrients vital for your skin, used alone or applied topically in a little cold pressed oil, provide magnificent *Monday Marinades*. In her exciting holistic book, *Ageless Aging,* Leslie Kenton describes a "skin cocktail," her very own Monday Marinade. It employs these intense healers right from the capsules with added evening primrose oil and an optional half-drop of Sandalwood. She says that "she will never want to be without it," that is until she "finds something better." Well, Leslie, check this one out! It includes lecithin, and an arsenal of essential oils.

JULIA'S INTENSIVE SKIN CARE RECIPE

To a tinted ½ ounce glass eye dropper bottle, available at your local drug store; or a tinted dropper bottle, from an aromatherapy supplier, add:

1 capsule of liquid lecithin or 420 mg phosphatidyl choline (available at your health food store)

1 drop of each of the following essential oils: Carrot Seed, Citrus, Neroli, Myrrh, Rose, Palma Rosa, Everlast, Frankincense, Rose Geranium, Lavender, Myrtle and Galbanum (the scent is divine).

1 teaspoon of rosehip or avocado oil, plus sufficient to fill the bottle (carrier oil) after all other ingredients are added.

2 caps ascorbyl palmitate (oil based vitamin C) yielding 300 mg of C

800 mg vitamin E (oil based).

7500 mg vitamin A (oil based)

1 cap Evening Primrose or Black Currant Seed oil.

Pierce the capsule of lecithin or phosphatidyl choline and squeeze the contents into the bottle. Add your essential oil blend into the bottle, allowing the lecithin and oils it to stand for about a half hour in the closed bottle. Note: Lecithin is very difficult to dissolve, but the essential oils will help. After the lecithin has "thinned," blend the mixture by gently rotating the bottle for a few minutes.

Empty the caps of ascorbyl palmitate into the teaspoon of carrier oil, working the white greasy powder into the oil. Add this mix into the bottle, and gently blend again. Pierce all remaining vitamin caps and add into the bottle. Blend.

Add your carrier oil (rosehip or avocado) to fill the bottle. Blend. Allow the preparation to stand in a cool dark place for several days before using.

To apply: Place a few drops into the palm of your hand. Dot a little on your neck and throat, cheeks, top of your lip and forehead. Working in an upward and outward direction begin at the base of your neck and gently massage the *marinade* into your skin. Stay at least a quarter of an inch from your eyes (the oils can sting). And, marinate!

If the mixture is too intense, dilute it further it by adding more of the carrier oil. If you feel you need it stronger, increase the percentage of essential oils. It is never necessary to use more than several drops at a time. For an all over body oil, the blend can be further diluted to a 2½ percent solution Note: As always, with sensitive skin, test first on a small area. To further customize your Marinade, see *Gourmet Ingredients* for additional selections or substitutions.

ET CETERAS

Some intensive marinades for a lazy Sunday or lonely Saturday when you, your skin and your nose have all the air to yourself include, straight from the container, plain **cod liver oil** or **extra virgin olive** (squeeze in a little Vitamin E). Spread all over the face. Soak as long as is comfortable. Reapply if needed.

And I confess to even trying . . . *yuck!* Sardine oil, straight from the can—not the vegetable packing oil, the straight *sild* with incredible results.

BUFFET STYLE "EYE-SINGS"

For beautiful eyes that are singing cheer,
These little hints will clear the blear.

Puffy "raccoon" eyes that spell **a-l-l-e-r-g-y, l-a-t-e n-i-g-h-t o-u-t, e-y-e s-t-r-a-i-n,** excess **f-l-u-i-d** or **t-o-x-i-n-s,** might try the following wrinkle, bag and dark circle removers as well as under-eye soothers.

THE EVER-READY The little blue gel or water filled masks that sit in the fridge.

THE OLD STANDBY Cool slices of Cucumber placed over the lids. Variation: first soak the slices in Milk.

TEA TIME Boil some water, pour it over a couple of tea bags, cool or refrigerate the bags. Enjoy the tea. Place cool moist tea bags over your eyes. Lie down and relax. Orange Pekoe works well, Chamomile, Fennel, Parsley or Eyebright will cleanse and remove dark circles, too.

UNSWELLIN' MELON A thin slice of Casaba Melon under each eye. (Pear works too). Lie down for 10 minutes.

POTATO MASH Grated potato in gauze pads.

SOFT SOAKS Cotton pads soaked in witch hazel or ice cold milk or buttermilk.

COMFREY-E Cold Comfrey tea bag compress, followed by a "touch" of vitamin E patted under your eyes.

TROPICAL TREASURE A Fig half placed over each eye will remove dark circles.

APPLE OF YOUR EYE Peel and grate an Apple, place in gauze pads, chill and apply.

EXOTIC EYES Soothing cold packs and compresses of 1 or 2 drops of the following in an 8 ounce bowl of distilled water, essential oil of Chamomile, Clary Sage, Geranium, Rose, and/or Fennel or a blend of any or all.

OFF BEAT FEET Place 6 drops of Peppermint oil in a cool foot bath and feel your eyes light up. There is a direct connection between tired sore feet and tired eyes.

SWEET SCENTED SLEEP Best rest for tired eyes. A drop or two of Lavender on your pillow.

TEMPLE MAGIC A drop of Lavender on the Temples relieves eye strain.

SALTY SOAK Another foot bath approach includes two soaks, one hot with Epsom salts (soak for 3 minutes), one cold (end with cold).

YEAST FEAST

½ tablespoon brewer's yeast or nutritional yeast
½ cup cold milk

Soak cotton pads with mixture. Place over your eyes. Removes bags too.

CUCUMBER SURPRISE

1 cucumber peeled and crushed
1 egg white
1 ounce witch hazel

Combine the egg white and witch hazel. Mix in the crushed cucumber. Add mixture into two pieces of cheese cloth or gauze pads. Place packs in freezer until firm (not frozen). Lie down with packs over eyes for about 10 minutes.

THE EYE LIFT

Preventing puffy eyes may mean cutting back salt intake, simply sleeping more, or tossing a too-heavy eye cream in the circular file. Chronic under eye bags may be genetic fatty deposits or the result of rough handling where the fabric of your skin has ruptured and the fatty tissue, no longer contained, spills out into pockets. For serious chronic bags surgery may be the only solution. But before you do anything radical try the following from the **Facelift Naturally** finger pressure program.

Using only the fleshy pads of your index fingers, press, the illustrated points in the following manner: With both fingers, one on either side of your face (the system is bilateral), very gently contact Point 1. Using no more than 4 pounds of pressure (check by pressing your fingers on your bathroom scale), slowly begin to press, gradually increasing the pressure. Do not rush.

Continue to press, proceeding very carefully. If, as you press, you experience discomfort, stop. Do not give yourself pain. Remain at a pleasing pressure for a slow count of 7, then release the pressure just as slowly. Keeping your fingers in light contact with your skin, remain touching for slow count of 5. Now, begin to press again, repeating the entire sequence for a total of three times.

Continue on to Point 2, and so on. When finished gently circle your eyes several times with a tapping motion, tapping lightly with the pads of your fingers.

This can be done once or twice a day to firm up the eyes, reduce puffiness and bags whatever the cause, and remove wrinkles. Caution: Do not touch any point that is irritated in any way; wait until it has healed before applying pressure.

"I"S-CREAM

The best creams for the eyes include a dab of lightweight vitamin E, or E diluted in a little cold pressed veggie oil; or rosehip seed oil with a drop or two of Myrtle and Rock Rose (Begin with a 2½% dilution).

The worst is any preparation containing mineral oil which can eventually rebound and dry, or lanolin which can cause sensitivities; neither penetrate the skin (molecular structure is too large), and both can cause puffiness. Test your vitamin E, as well, some types can also cause reactions.

"EYE"-DEAS!

Hint: Even if your skin is oily-oily, your eyes can still lack sufficient lubrication. Be sure to moisturize and apply an eye cream or oil or lotion.

Hint: When touching the eye area, always "fingerprint" makeup, lotions, or creams onto the skin, rolling the finger gently, and circle from the inner corner out, on the upper lid and the outer corner in on the under eye.

Hint: To help repair damaged under eye tissue, nutritional help suggests protein, Vitamin C and organic silica.

Hint: For various eye problems, **Eyebright** capsules taken orally or prepared as a tea or eyewash is the herb of choice. Cayenne, Bayberry Bark and Red Raspberry Leaves **taken internally** as teas are also traditional approaches.

Hint: To tighten under eyes, before making up, after washing, coat lightly with Buttermilk.

Hint: Always sunscreen the delicate eye area with special sunblocks for the eyes. Wear wide brimmed hats when exposed to the sun.

Hint: No joke, **Carrot Juice,** really does make you see better. High in beta carotene (provitamin A), a lack of which (even a slight lack) can cause your eyes to tire quickly, to be light sensitive and have dry lids. Other necessary nutrients for bright eyes include: the B-complex, C, E and zinc.

IV.
SPECIALITIES OF
THE HOUSE:
SKIN TIGHTENERS

An amazing trio of dynamite recipes, used regularly, the following will delay and/or reverse signs of facial aging. And—if you are already practicing **Facelift Naturally,** *the following is "icing" on the crouton.*

FRESH FROM THE CRISPER

THE "FREEZE LIFT"

The best way to revive a wilted romaine, celery stalk, or carrot stick is to place it in ice water. This little trick has saved many a salad, and, would you believe, many a face, as well. The taut rosy faces of winter are ready examples. And rumor has it that certain movie stars always take the frigid plunge before going in front of the camera. Whether or not there's truth to the rumor (my guess is yes), the method certainly works. I first encountered the idea some twenty years ago in a book by Jessica Krane, a wonderfully intelligent, remarkably innovative woman intent on saving her skin. Jessica wrote, "... for almost four years I have frozen my face every day— well over 1,000 times in all. . . . At this writing, my facial skin tightly adheres to its structure . . . perhaps more tightly now than when I was under twenty." (She never would tell her age.) She also cautioned that if she stopped her facial freeze for only one day, she noticed the difference.

The *crisping* unquestionably works. I saw an immediate difference when I tried it myself. Also, it took less than a week to notice smaller pores, a detectable facial glow and definite overall tightness. Recently a woman informed me that she remembered her mother rubbing an ice cube over her face before retiring at night, and her face was tight and smooth well into her seventies.

It has been suggested that facial freezing might blemish the skin or injure the delicate facial capillaries. My skin tends to the sensitive side, but I'm signed up for life. However, if you have super-sensitive skin when water of any temperature is a problem, then, of course, don't attempt this. Or, if you have a cold or sinus condition, you might want to think twice. Jessica and her students had no difficulties, she said. In fact, she noted that the procedure seemed to add to her overall resistance. I have found the same.

THE PREPARATION

Since you will be splashing your face with ice water, the best time to practice your freeze lift, or facial *crisping,* is before, during or after a shower or bath. A creative time saver might suggest floating a bowl of ice, or ice water in the bath. While a more leisurely approach is to stand in front of a sink filled with about 30 regular ice cubes to a quart and a half of water.

With your hair pulled back from your clean, clean face, apply cream or oil. This is protection for your skin and provides a basis for the freezing. Sensitive skins should apply heavy creams. Cotton lined rubber gloves will protect your hands.

THE CRISPING

The first day: Begin with five splashes of ice water to the cheekbones. Next, five splashes to the chin area, five below the chin, and five to the neck (twenty splashes). Repeat once more (forty splashes in all).

The second day: Begin as the first day, but repeat to eighty splashes total. As your face reaches freezing, it will become numb and start to glow. At this time, add more ice water to the areas that need extra firming. To finish, sensitive skins may choose to gently press-dry their faces with a soft towel. Hardier skins may opt for further stimulation and toning with the use of a **strigil** (an instrument of Roman—*as in the baths*—origin), employed by Jessica to reduce facial flabbiness.

THE STRIGIL

Making a strigil: Using a new, fairly coarse kitchen sponge (the kind that is about 4" × 6"), cut an inch-and-a-quarter wide section from the long side of the sponge, so that you have a strip that is 1¼" × 6". This provides an instrument long enough to fit comfortably in your hand and narrow enough for use on your face.

USING THE STRIGIL

Still in the middle of "crisping," face totally devoid of feeling (after 80–100 splashes of ice water), assume the following facial expression: first purse your lips to whistle, simultaneously force your chin down. This opens your lips slightly— too wide to whistle, but just open enough to allow a deep throaty utterance that sounds like "woo." This facial pose not only holds your skin taut, smoothing out lines and wrinkles, but stretches underlying muscles, helping to firm and tone the face. An exercise, by the way, that can be repeated in sets of 50 at intervals during the day with obvious benefit.

Now, strigil in hand, omitting the forehead and under eye area, begin at the cheekbones and tap over the areas indicated in the illustration. **Facelift Naturally** practitioners will recognize them instantly. Work down one side of your face, slowly and lightly brush-tapping each point with a sharp, but gentle, touch. When finished work down the other side. Having gently stimulated your face, gingerly press-dry with a soft towel. Add cream below the eyes and upper cheekbones.

THE "CRISPER" SHORT CUT

There are just some situations that call for freezing on the run. So, the following less comprehensive program for critical situations might be considered. For instance, a very important friend calls. You're totally wilted and have exactly 10 minutes to *be crisped and dressed*. Or, you are at a party or function where it is impossible to "splash." But you are exhausted and you know that your face has absolutely "had it."

Quick, grab a glass. Pop in a couple of cubes. There is usually a bar, a fridge, or, at the very least, a cooler with a bag of ice nearby. Slip into the rest room. Put a towel (paper is okay) around your neck. Place an ice cube in each hand and with lightning speed gently glide in little circles over your cheeks and neck (ladies, makeup and all). Do this several times. For that all-over wakeup feeling, include the back of the ears. Blot. With a few touch-ups, you're good for the rest of the party. Note: Hold the cubes under running water for a few seconds to make sure there are no internal stresses that will make the cubes pop while you are running them over your face. The experience can be quite startling. To be on the safe side, close your eyes as you apply them to your face. For super tightening, if your hair style will allow, rub the cubes over your hairline, as well.

THE CAESAR SUPREME (HOLD THE ANCHOVIES)

AKA: THE INCREDIBLE FACE LIFTING, SKIN TONING, MUSCLE FIRMING FACE MASK THAT REALLY WORKS!

When you need to have every radish, cucumber slice, tomato and onion ring in place and be "dressed" to kill, the following recipe can be whipped up in seconds ... Requires about 15 minutes to one half hour to "take" and can hold up to 8 hours. You may want to try it, two or three times weekly, at first. Then once a week should do it. Brown spots and wrinkles will lighten, circulation and all over firmness improve. Rejuvenating effects are cumulative.

The **Caesar Supreme** relies on basically two main ingredients Albumen and Aloe Vera. Also, some very helpful additional options are listed. All ingredients can be found at, or ordered by, your local health food store.

MAIN INGREDIENTS

Albumen in the form of 100% egg protein powder, a food supplement to which bromelin and/or papain are sometimes added. Both bromelin and papain are protein digesting enzymes that will help to dissolve dead skin tissue. Also, since the powder is a food supplement, vanilla flavor is, generally, added. One brand sold in gyms and health food stores is produced by Beverly International. If you prefer 100% dried egg white with no additives, you may wish to contact Jim Younger, c/o THE GYM, 2055 Glacier Lane, Plymouth, MN, 55447; phone: 612-553-0171. One pound containers sell for about $14.00. The protein powder is very cost effective (a little goes a long way); it's clean (no leftover refrigerator mess) and the powder can be premixed with any or all of the listed options. Fresh egg white may also be used, see below.

Aloe vera in liquid form. Prepared aloe products of high quality are necessary. Many varieties, even in health food stores are diluted and ineffective for this purpose. Brands of excellent quality are: Forever Living Products "aloe activator," (3 oz. / $12.00) and Metaloe (Metabolic Technology) (check your phone book for local distributors), Salute (health food stores), Zia Cosmetics Sea Tonic and Aloe Toner, 1-800-334-SKIN, 8 oz. for $12.95.

NOTE: Read labels when you shop for aloe products. Some contain potassium sorbate or sorbic acid that can cause redness and burning lasting up to 45 minutes if you have a sensitivity to these preservatives.

OPTIONAL INGREDIENTS

To be added to the dry albumen prior to mixing with aloe:

A pinch of kelp (seaweed found in crushable tablets and powder) or spirulina—both add mineral nutrients from the sea.

A dash of skin soothing Chamomile and/or Comfrey (dry herbs, or see below for essential oils).

A pinch or two of fullers earth, pascalite clay or corn starch (okay for all skin types).

Essential oils to be added to the Aloe prior to mixing with the albumen. 1 or 2 drops of one or a blend of the following essential oils: Jasmine, Neroli, Sandalwood, Frankincense, Myrrh, Cistus, Rose Geranium, Lavender, Ylang-Ylang,

Rose (extremely expensive; if this oil is not expensive, it is not the real thing. Use only genuine essential oils.)

Note: When adding essential oils, add no more than the recipe requires. These are very concentrated, powerful oils that penetrate deeply into the skin. If you prefer a blend of oils, blend first, then add 1 or 1 drops of the blend to your "dressing." For a more specific explanation of what the oils do and other options for particular skin conditions, see Gourmet Ingredients. If you have difficulty in locating a particular oil, or prefer to buy in quantity, distributors are listed in Essential Oils: Resourses.

Culinary purists may opt for fresh Egg White and/or Aloe Vera. If you opt for fresh Aloe, Marinading Mature, you may want to mix in a little purified Sea Water (available in health food stores), *in addition to the listed options. If you enjoy cooking and saving money, experimenting with the proportions and mixing up your own masks can be fun. If not, masks can be purchased ready-made from Zia Cosmetics and Forever Living Products, among others.*

THE RECIPE

1½ teaspoons albumen (with optional kelp or spirulina, fuller's earth, pascalite clay, dry herbs and/or cornstarch added).

1½ teaspoons aloe, more or less (with optional drop or two of essential oils or blends).

Slowly add the aloe to the albumen until you have a mixture the consistency of a thin lotion. Using a "blusher" brush, apply evenly to a clean face. Beginning low on the neck, brush in an upward and outward motion. Cover the throat, behind the ears and the face, taking care to avoid the eye area. Lie down with a towel under your head to catch any drips and relax. Allow the mask to dry and tighten for 15 minutes (dry or sensitive skins); and up to 30 minutes (normal skin), taking care to keep your facial muscles still as the mask tightens.

To remove: first soften with a dampened face cloth or towel, then gently rinse (20–30 splashes) with warm water. If there is itching from the stimulation, simply press the area with your finger, or apply an ice cube; avoid scratching. Apply toner and moisturizer as usual. Wait for 10 minutes to apply makeup.

THE YOUTHFUL
YEAST YUMMY

A recipe that dreams are made of. Worth more than its weight in *crudites,* this crowd pleaser works intense magic at "intimate" dinner parties. Not the most scent-uous or tasty dressing but the results are superb. In minutes, you "emerge," skin stretched tautly over your face, fine lines washed down the kitchen drain. The effects hold for hours. Don't waste this one if you are dining alone.

An intense once-a-week-workout for all skin types, except very sensitive and rosacea complexions, that's jam-packed with vitamins, minerals, RNA, DNA, SOD and nutritional "face foods," the Youthful Yeast Yummy increases facial circulation and is a catalyst for healthy cell reproduction. Used long-term, a definite wrinkle preventor. Following are two versions.

Note: If your complexion is OverSeasoned Sensitive, this may be too much for you. The mask is very stimulating.

VERSION #1

Here, moisturizing honey teams up with acid-balancing cider vinegar and softening vegetable oil to enhance the nutritious yeast formulation.

½ teaspoon brewer's or nutritional yeast
Enough water to barely dissolve the yeast, add by drops
1 tablespoon honey
1 tablespoon vegetable oil
¼ teaspoon apple cider vinegar

Dissolve the yeast in the water. Blend with the remaining ingredients. Before applying, oil face and neck. Note: Brewer's yeast can irritate the skin of the neck; avoid your neck area if this is a problem. Also, avoid your delicate eye area.

VERSION #2

More drying than the above recipe, this version includes aloe juice which is soothing and healing for minor skin irritations and blemishes, as well as acne and can be used up to three times weekly for clearing blemishes. When clear, once a week will do. Also fantastic for maintaining unblemished skin.

2 tablespoons (heaping) powdered brewer's yeast, or nutritional yeast
1 tablespoon aloe juice
1 egg white

Mix to form a thick paste. Before applying, lightly oil your face and neck area. When applying, avoid your delicate eye area. Then, starting from the base of your neck, moving upward and outward, apply the mask, covering every pore **except** your delicate eye area.

Turn on soothing music, TV or a relaxation tape. Lie down. Keep your face muscles absolutely still. Marinate for about

30–45 minutes. In about 10 minutes, as the mask begins to "cook," you'll start to feel a tingling in your skin. After the mask has hardened, use a dampened face cloth to "crack" the mask, then flood the face, splashing with tepid water. Finally, use a dampened cloth to remove all traces. Splash with tepid water. Apply your moisturizer.

When you look in the mirror, your skin will be flushed and red. This is due to the restriction-stimulation effect of the mask as it dries. The lower dermal layer is stimulated to rejuvenating activity, while the upper epidermis is restricted, tightening the pores. In a few minutes, the redness will subside, leaving you with a fabulous recipe that you'll continue to use at every dinner party.

V.

PLANT FOOD PLUS:
FEEDING YOUR SKIN—
FROM WITHIN

> Sunlight and water makes the salad grow,
> With fertile soil to nourish.
> Dewy complexions, sunscreened cheeks,
> Let's see what makes faces flourish.

Aware of the importance and dangers of sunlight and our need for water, healthy skin, glowing with vitality, requires feeding from the "roots" up. Nutrition is a major consideration.

PROTEIN

Next to water, protein is the most plentiful substance in skin. About 27 percent, protein is the glue that holds your skin together. Collagen is protein. Elastin is protein. Enzymes and hormones are protein, and skin-protecting antibodies are protein. So forget all the fruit-only and liquid-only diets— without adequate protein your facial skin will sag down around your ankles.

How much protein is enough? The daily requirement of a 170 pound man involved in light work is about 30 grams. With heavier work or in times of stress extra protein is needed. Too much protein can cause a fluid imbalance or lead to calcium depletion in your bones.

It is important that your body takes in complete proteins.

During digestion, the large protein molecules are broken down into amino acids, which are the "building blocks" needed for all the proteins responsible for the growth and repair of healthy skin.

Your body needs approximately 22 amino acids in a specific pattern to make a human protein, eight of which cannot be produced by the body. These eight are called the "essential amino acids," because it is essential that you obtain all of these from your diet. If just one is missing, even temporarily, protein synthesis will either stop or become low, because all of the amino acids will fall in the same proportion as the low or missing amino acid. To properly synthesize protein for use in your body, all the needed amino acids must be present.

Some foods contain all the essential amino acids and are called complete proteins. They are found in most meat, fish and dairy products. Incomplete proteins are mostly found in vegetables and fruits. Complete proteins are formed, however, when beans combine with corn, wheat, nuts, rice, seeds or cheese; and, when brown rice combines with beans, nuts, seeds or cheese. Cornmeal fortified with the amino acid L-lysine makes a complete protein. Soybean products (tofu, soybean milk) are complete proteins. Strict vegetarians, however, must supplement with vitamin B12, a vitamin that is found only in meat.

Supplementation with free form amino acids and/or digestive enzymes are helpful if you have difficulty digesting or assimilating protein. See also *Anti-Aging Anti-Oxidants*. *For* a breakfast drink, or a meal, a protein rich recipe is ...

THE SKIN SHAKE

6 ounces nonfat milk
1 tablespoon protein powder
1 tablespoon nutritional yeast powder (B vitamins)
½ tablespoon blackstrap molasses (minerals and B vitamins)
2–3 tablespoons acidophilus to promote healthy digestive flora
1 tablespoon granulated lecithin to break down cholesterol
    bumps under the skin
Add some strawberries and/or a banana or fruit to taste
A few ice cubes and blend until frothy

CARBOHYDRATES

"Carbs" are the body's chief source of fuel. They are the sugars and starches that are burned for energy. If no carbs are around to burn, your body will use your protein supply depleting your skin. Eat only complex carbohydrates found in fresh fruits, vegetables, beans, and natural whole grains.

ESSENTIAL FATTY ACIDS

Also known as polyunsaturates, vitamin F or EFAs, *essential* means these fats are diet dependent and cannot be manufactured in the body. Necessary fuel, the EFA daily requirement is about 10 to 20 percent of total calorie intake. A medium for supplying oil soluble vitamins to the body, EFAs are recommended to lower blood pressure and reduce heart disease and stroke. A diet lacking polyunsaturates will result in dry scaly skin. Sources include: grains, nuts, vegetables and seeds, also cold water fish, such as salmon, cod, haddock and mackerel (fish oils have been known to improve psoriasis). See *A Splash of Oil; Anti-Aging Antioxidants*.

FIBER

Found in many foods, fiber helps to prevent disorders that range from constipation to cancer. It helps lower cholesterol levels, stabilize blood sugar and prevent obesity. *Insoluble fiber plus water scrubs up the inner you, reflecting in a clean clear complexion.* Because of refined foods, the American diet lacks fiber; figures of colon cancer are growing yearly.

There are actually seven forms, but two basic types of fiber, **insoluble** which makes up the walls of plants, these speed food through the intestines absorbing a great deal of water along the way. Brans, apple skins are examples. And, *soluble* fiber, in the form of pectin, slows food absorption, is excellent for diabetics. Removing toxins and metals, it is useful also in radiation therapy. Pectin is found in apples, carrots, beets, bananas, cabbage, citrus, dried peas and okra. If taking supplemental fiber, be sure to start with small amounts and increase your intake slowly. Much water will be absorbed by the fiber, so increase your water intake.

THE SKIN-VITES

Extremely important to good skin and overall good health, very few vitamins can be produced in your system and must be supplied by diet.

VITAMIN A

Free-radical fighter vitamin A *helps to maintain soft smooth, young-looking skin. A deficiency in this vitamin is exhibited in rough, wrinkled, goosebump-like scaly skin.*

Also known as retinol, after the retina of the eye which has a particular need for this vitamin, "A" protects against night blindness and other eye problems, guarding the mucous membranes of your nose, mouth, throat and lungs, as well as reducing your susceptibility to infection and, most probably, lung cancer.

Oil soluble, vitamin A is stored in the liver, where high supplemental doses can accumulate. In adults, more than 85,000 IU a day quickly becomes toxic, resulting in nausea, dizziness, headaches, vomiting, or worse—it can be lethal. *Too much "A" can cause dry, itchy skin and lips, loss of hair, and, possibly, a yellowish tint to the skin.*

Under a doctor's care, high doses of 100,000 IU are used for treating acne, oily skin and large pores. This dosage should not be taken for more than a few weeks. Mostly used in doses of 15,000 to 35,000 IU with 25 mg of supplemental harmless, beta carotene or "pro-vitamin A," that can be converted to vitamin A in the intestine and then stored in the liver, the remainder circulates in the blood. 25 mg of beta carotene provides 40,000 IU of potential vitamin A activity. How much beta carotene you absorb depends on the kind and amount of fats you have eaten.

Vitamin A and/or carotene is found highly concentrated in fish-liver oils; it is found also in animal livers and green vegetables, yellow and orange vegetables. Cod liver oil or vitamin A should not be taken in large amounts in pill form by anyone with liver problems. Pregnant women should not take over 25,000 IU. Diabetics and hyperthyroid individuals cannot convert beta carotene into "A." Destroyed by heat and light, store this vitamin in a cool dark place. See also *Anti-Aging Antioxidants*.

THE "Bs"

Coenzymes, the "Bs" are important for skin maintenance, care of the eyes, hair, liver, mouth and muscle tone. Maintaining healthy nerves, they are used to treat depression or anxiety. Very involved in energy production, these water soluble vitamins are a team; one should not be taken without the entire complex. Although, for specific problems, individual Bs may be added into the group.

B1 (THIAMINE)

B1 is needed for circulation and rosy complexions, production of hydrochloric acid, blood formation, carbohydrate metabolism, and help for the nervous system. If you have a sweet tooth, like a drink more than now and then, exercise intensely, or use oral contraceptives, you may be a candidate for thiamine supplementation. Good sources for thiamine are: pork, organ meats, poultry, oysters, egg yolks, brewer's yeast, whole grains, wheat germ, oatmeal, lima beans, soy beans, brown rice, Brussels sprouts, most nuts, plums, dried prunes and raisins.

B2 (RIBOFLAVIN)

Very important for your skin's balance. B2 deficiencies may be seen as cracked and chapped lips or cracks at the corners to an excessively oily face with scaliness around the mouth and nose. Involved in many bodily functions, B2 should be supplemented by women taking oral contraceptives and those who exercise a great deal. This vitamin is easily destroyed by light cooking, antibiotics and alcohol. Sources for B2 are: meat, poultry, eggs, cheese, milk, yogurt, beans, spinach, whole grains, and mushrooms.

B3 (NIACIN, NIACINAMIDE, NICOTINIC ACID)

Necessary for circulation and oxygenation of healthy skin, B3 is important for the functioning of the nervous system, the metabolism of carbohydrates, fats and proteins and the production of digestive hydrochloric acid as well. Sources are: beef, broccoli, carrots, cheese, cereals, corn flour, eggs, fish, liver, milk, pork, potatoes, tomatoes and whole wheat.

Caution: A usually harmless flush may occur after taking as little as 50 mg of niacin, including a red rash, and tingling sensation. If you have broken capillaries, acne rosacea, thin or sensitive skin, avoid niacin supplementation. High amounts should be used with discretion by pregnant women, those who suffer with gout, peptic ulcers, glaucoma, liver disease and diabetes.

PANTOTHENIC ACID (B5)

Pantothenic acid, known as the "antistress" vitamin, assists in tissue metabolism and plays a role in the production of vital steroids and cortisone in the adrenal glands. *Deficiency may result in gray hair, stunted growth, dermatitis,* numbness in the fingers and toes and personality changes. Too much can cause diarrhea and edema. Good sources: beef, pork, liver, kidney, salt-water fish, eggs, pork, beans, fresh dark green veggies, and whole wheat.

B6 (PYRIDOXINE)

Involved in more bodily functions than any one nutrient, B6 affects both physical and mental health. Aiding in the production of hydrochloric acid and the absorption of fats and protein, *Pyridoxine also assists in the formation of red blood cells, protein and your skin's keratin. B6 also maintains your sodium and potassium balance. If your skin type is OverRipe Fruit, consider B6 for water retention problems.*

Needed for the nervous system, B6 is necessary for normal brain activity and for DNA/RNA synthesis, the nucleic acids that provide all the genetic instruction for cell reproduction and normal growth. Ranging from cancer prevention to inhibiting fatty deposits around the heart, Pyridoxine activates many enzymes and is involved in B12 absorption.

Deficiencies may be instrumental in anemia, cracks in mouth corners, over oily skin, scaling, lesions, and a reduction in the skin's ability to fight off infection. Carpal tunnel syndrome is also linked to a B6 deficiency. Linked strongly to protein assimilation, the more protein you eat, the more B6 you need. If you are taking oral contraceptives, antidepressants, estrogen or are under stress, a lack of B6 can result in mild depression.

All foods contain some B6. The highest sources are: lean meats, poultry, fish and eggs; brewer's yeast, carrots, peas, spinach, sunflower seeds, walnuts and wheat germ. Lesser amounts are found in avocado, cabbage and cantaloupe, bananas, beans, blackstrap molasses, brown rice and whole grains.

B12 (CYANOCOBALAMIN)

Pale lemon yellow skin, numbness and tingling in the toes and fingers, loss of balance, memory loss, hallucinations, eye and digestive disorders, anemia and all over *weakness can signal a lack of B12*. An aid in the *formation and longevity of your cells,* B12 is also required for good digestion, food absorption, protein synthesis and the metabolism of fats and carbohydrates. B12 prevents nerve damage, while maintaining fertility, normal development and growth. Older adults and those with digestive disorders may suffer from a B12 deficiency due to an inability to absorb the vitamin. Vegetarians are also at risk, since B12 is found only in animal sources. Anti-gout medications, anticoagulants and potassium supplements may block B12 absorption.

Highest amounts occur in cheese (particularly blue), seafood: clams, herring, mackerel; kidney, liver, eggs, milk, and tofu.

BIOTIN

Needed for healthy skin and hair, biotin aids in cell growth, the production of fatty acids and the metabolism of "carbs," fats, and proteins. It may also prevent hair loss in some men. Needed for the utilization of the entire B-complex, biotin initiates healthy sweat glands, bone marrow and nerve tissue. Deficiencies of biotin are rare, because it can be produced from foods in the intestines. The consumption of large amounts of raw egg white can cause problems, since raw egg whites contain the protein ovidin, which combines with biotin in the intestines and depletes the body of this vitamin. Deficiencies can also occur with the use of sulfa drugs and some antibiotics, also the consumption of rancid fats or saccharin. Good sources of biotin are found in meat, liver, poultry, salt-water fish (sardines), milk, egg yolk, brewer's yeast, whole grains and green beans.

CHOLINE

Aiding in hormone and lecithin production, very important for healthy skin, choline is also needed for nerve transmission, the metabolism of fat and cholesterol, gall bladder regulation and liver function. Deficiencies may contribute to fatty build-up in the liver, memory impairment, brain dysfunction, Parkinson's disease and tardive dyskinesia. Good sources are: meat, milk, egg yolks, legumes, and whole grains.

FOLIC ACID

"Brain food," folic acid works best when combined with B12. An energy-giver, aiding in the formation of red blood cells, folic acid is very important in the treatment of folic acid anemia. Instrumental in synthesizing genetic material, folic acid also offsets pigmentary changes. *Deficiencies can be seen in brownish skin pigmentation, dull and premature gray hair*, and a sore red tongue. Too much can cause irritability and sleeplessness.

Folic acid in significant quantities is found in beef, chicken, lamb, pork, liver and organ meats, salmon, tuna and cheese; brewer's yeast, bran, barley, brown rice, lentils, wheat germ, whole wheat and whole grains; green leafy veggies, broccoli and root veggies; and oranges.

INOSITOL

Important for hair growth, inositol helps to prevent hardening of the arteries. An aid to fat removal from the liver this vitamin is important in the *formation of lecithin* and in the metabolism of fat and cholesterol.

Found in meats, milk, whole grains, vegetables and fruits, heavy caffeine consumption may cause shortages of inositol.

VITAMIN C (Ascorbic Acid)

Vital for every tissue in your body including teeth, cartilage, muscle and bone, a shortage of vitamin C will show up very quickly in your skin, especially if you are older, smoke or take oral contraceptives, aspirin, steroids and/or tetracycline. *Without C, collagen can't be produced and your facial skin will be back down around your ankles. If you've noticed a slowdown in your healing time, puffy eyes when you awaken, swelling in your legs, bleeding gums, and/or rough, discolored, dry skin with obvious follicles, you are very likely deficient in this water soluble vitamin* that is easily expelled through the urine and needs to be constantly replenished.

Vitamin C, one of the free-radical scavenging "ACEs," enhances immunity, protecting against the harmful effects of pollution, infection and cancer. Guarding against blood clots, this producer of antistress hormones aids in the production of interferon, is needed in the metabolism of folic acid, and the amino acids tyrosine and phenylalanine.

Working synergistically with vitamin E, the protecting effects are greater. "E" scavenges for the dangerous free radicals in the cell membrane, while "C" breaks down the free radical chain in the biologic fluids. Together "C" and "E" extend antioxidant activity greatly.

A breakthrough in vitamin C has come in the form of Ester C polysorbate (esterified C), which is good news for sufferers of chronic illnesses like cancer and AIDS. With Ester C, white blood cell levels of "C" are increased four times over the average ascorbic acid "C" and only one third the amount is excreted in the urine—a major boon to the immune system.

Good sources of "C" include green vegetables (beet and turnip greens, broccoli, Brussels sprouts, kale, mustard greens, Swiss chard, watercress, collards, mustard greens, parsley, green peppers, spinach, green peas); onions, avocados, citrus fruits (lemons, oranges, grapefruit), tomatoes, strawberries, mangos, currants, papaya, persimmons, pineapple and rose hips. See also *Anti-Aging Antioxidants*.

Diabenase (diabetic drug) and sulfa drugs may be less effective when taken with vitamin C. Large amounts of this vitamin can cause a false negative reading when testing for occult blood in the stool. Pregnant women should keep dosages of "C" at 5,000 mg a day or less.

BIOFLAVONOIDS

If you have "broken capillaries," bioflavonoids are for you. They protect and preserve the structure of the capillary walls. Sometimes referred to as vitamin P, bioflavonoids are not vitamins in the true sense. They are considered part of the C-complex. Enhancing the absorption of vitamin C, they should be taken together. Not produced by the body, bioflavonoids must be supplied by the diet. Used extensively in sports related injuries, bioflavonoids relieve pain, swelling and bruising.

If you look under your orange, lemon, or grapefruit peel, you will find a bioflavonoid in the white pulp. Also found, in peppers, buckwheat (kasha), black currents, apricots, cherries, grapes, prunes and rosehips.

VITAMIN D

Needed for the absorption and utilization of calcium and phosphorus, *fat soluble vitamin D is made on the skin when exposed to sunlight. Just by exposing the face and arms fifteen minutes a day the need for vitamin D is met.* Although "D" is found in many foods, it is not fully activated until it undergoes conversion first by the liver and then by the kidney. People with kidney or liver disease are at higher risk for osteoporosis, unless exposed to sunlight.

Also considered an antioxidant and anticarcinogen, *vitamin D has some sunscreening properties, and may be instrumental in regulating skin pigmentation.* Deficiencies can result in depression, noted where winters are long; muscle spasms and twitching; and soft fragile deformed bones.

Besides the ultraviolet radiation of the sun, good sources include fish liver oils: cod liver, halibut liver, fatty salt-water fish: salmon, sardines, tuna, herring, dairy products fortified with vitamin D, eggs (yolk), butter, alfalfa, oatmeal, sweet potatoes, and vegetable oils.

Vitamin D should not be taken without calcium and doses of over 65,000 IU over a period of time may cause toxicity. Thiazide diuretics upset the calcium/"D" balance. Intestinal, liver and gallbladder malfunctions interfere with absorption, as does the use of some cholesterol-lowering drugs, antacids, mineral oil and cortisone.

VITAMIN E

One of the vitamin ACEs, high doses of "E" produce a photoprotective effect, shielding from UV (ultraviolet) radiation, and reducing sun induced redness. Vitamin E retards aging, prevents cataracts and may prevent "age spots", as well. Tissue repairing "E," topically applied, acts as a moisturizer and sunscreen that also reduces some wound scarring. "E" is an antioxidant that prevents cancer and cardiovascular disease, preventing cell damage by inhibiting lipid peroxidation (rancid fats) in the body and the formation of free radicals. It helps form red blood cells, improves circulation, repairs tissue, is used in treating fibrocystic breasts, menopausal problems (hot flushes and cramping) and PMS (premenstrual syndrome), promotes normal clotting and works synergistically with vitamins A and C increasing vitamin A absorption.

Sources for "E" include nuts, seeds and legumes, dry beans, whole grains, wheat germ, oatmeal, brown rice, cornmeal, desiccated liver and organ meats, eggs and milk, sweet potatoes, dark leafy greens, and cold pressed vegetable oils. See *A Splash of Oil.*

If you avoid all fats in your diet, you are a candidate for "E" deficiency. If you are low in zinc, the "E" levels in your blood will also be low. "E" and iron should not be taken at the same time. Use only low doses of "E" if you suffer from diabetes, rheumatic heart disease or an overactive thyroid. If you have high blood pressure and wish to supplement, start

first with very low doses, increasing slowly to the desired dose.
Consult first with your doctor. See also *Anti-Aging Antioxidants.*

VITAMIN K

*Deriving its name from the German **Koagulation**, vitamin
"K" is necessary for skin healing and normal blood clotting.*
Manufactured by the intestinal flora, vitamin K converts glucose into glycogen for storage in the liver and may also prevent osteoporosis. When taking antibiotics, intestinal flora are
killed and supplements of "K" may be necessary. If you
bruise easily, you may be deficient in vitamin K. Megadoses,
however, can accumulate and cause flushing and sweating.
Pregnant women, in the last weeks should avoid large doses
of synthetic "K," since this could result in a toxic effect on
the newborn.

"K" is found in broccoli, dark leafy greens, Brussels
sprouts, cabbage and cauliflower, alfalfa and soybeans, oats,
rye and wheat, liver and egg yolks, blackstrap molasses and
safflower oil.

COENZYME Q10

*A vitamin-like substance resembling vitamin E, but perhaps
an even more powerful antioxidant, Coenzyme Q10 is crucial
for the immune system and retards aging.* Also known as ubi-
quinone, CoQ10 diminishes with age and should be supplemented. According to the New England Institute, CoQ10 alone
is effective in reducing mortality rates in experimental animals
afflicted with tumors and leukemia. Used as a treatment for
heart disease and high blood pressure in Japan, research has
proven that Coenzyme Q10 helps allergy and asthma sufferers
and those who have respiratory problems. It is also helpful in
the treatment of brain anomalies such as those associated with

schizophrenia and Alzheimer's disease, aging, obesity, candidiasis, MS (multiple sclerosis), periodontal disease and diabetes. It may be a major step in the control of cancer and AIDS because of its huge benefit to the immune system.

When taking CoQ10, take care to purchase only the purist form. It is bright yellow and has almost no taste in the powdered form. Store away from heat and light.

Food sources containing the largest quantities of CoQ10 are mackerel, salmon and sardines. See also *Anti-Aging Antioxidants*.

"SKIN"ERALS

Minerals, like vitamins, act as coenzymes, and are needed for the body to carry on its many activities: form blood and bone, maintain healthy nerve function, and are needed for the composition of body fluids.

There are two types of minerals, bulk and trace. The bulk minerals are required in larger quantities than the trace minerals of which only minute amounts are needed. Bulk minerals include: calcium, magnesium, sodium, potassium and phosphorus. Trace minerals, though small quantities are utilized, are very important for good health. They include, boron, zinc, iron, copper, manganese, chromium, selenium and iodine. Basically stored in bone and muscle, it is possible to overdose on large quantities of minerals.

Some minerals are available in chelated form; these are more readily absorbed due to the attached protein molecule that acts as a transport to the bloodstream. Taken with meals, minerals are usually chelated automatically during digestion in the stomach.

Due to the nature of mineral absorption by the body, it is necessary to take a balanced mineral supplement, since if you take too much of one mineral it may deplete the body of another. For instance, if you take more zinc than necessary, it will deplete your body of copper; too much calcium can affect magnesium. Also, fiber will decrease absorption. If you are taking supplemental fiber, take your mineral at a different time.

BORON

Needed for calcium uptake, boron is not usually deficient in most people. Elderly people, however, due to difficulty with calcium absorption, may benefit from 2–3 mg a day. A study on postmenopausal women showed that within eight days of supplementing with 3 mg of boron, 40% less calcium, and one third less magnesium was excreted in the urine.

Good sources include leafy veggies, fruits, nuts and grains.

If supplementing, never take more than 3 mg daily.

CALCIUM

The most abundant mineral in the body, 98% of calcium is found in the teeth and bones. Important in the formation and maintenance of healthy teeth and bones, as well as maintenance, calcium is also necessary for a regular heartbeat, the transmission of nerve impulses, muscle growth and function, blood clotting, the prevention of cancer. Calcium participates in the structuring of DNA/RNA, and is involved in activating several enzymes.

Deficiencies result in osteoporosis, irregular heart beat or palpitations, muscle cramps, *split nails, eczema,* high blood pressure and cholesterol levels, tooth decay, insomnia, rickets, numbness in the arms and/or legs, aching joints and rheumatoid arthritis.

Natural food sources for calcium include: dairy foods including goat's milk, sardines and salmon with bones, seafood, leafy greens. Also found in almonds, asparagus, blackstrap molasses, brewer's yeast, broccoli, cabbage, carob, figs, filbert's, oats, prunes, sesame seeds and tofu.

Who needs more calcium? Female athletes, menopausal and postmenopausal women (estrogen promotes the deposit of calcium in the bone), pregnant women, nursing mothers, smokers, alcohol and caffeine drinkers and people who are stressed.

What inhibits calcium absorption? Soybeans, cooked spinach, kale, rhubarb, beet greens, almonds, cashews, chard and cocoa (casual consumption shouldn't hurt), insufficient vitamin D, or excess phosphorus (average American diet, high in meats, refined grains and soft drinks), excess magnesium, excess zinc, iron taken at the same time (neutralizes both), and Tums (neutralizes stomach acids needed to break down calcium for assimilation).

Who shouldn't supplement? Anyone with kidney stones or kidney disease, anyone on Verapamil, a calcium channel blocker for the heart.

Is your calcium supplement good? It is if it breaks down in a glass of warm water within twenty-four hours. It isn't if it's D1-calcium-phosphate in a multimineral supplement (this form of calcium interferes with the absorption of the multisupplement.

CHROMIUM (GTF)

Involved in the metabolism of glucose, chromium GTF (glucose tolerance factor) is important for energy, while maintaining stable blood sugar levels through the proper use of insulin.

Coronary heart disease patients will show a low plasma level of chromium. The average American is chromium deficient, two out of three being either hypoglycemic or prehypoglycemic or diabetic, according to researchers. Cause results from a diet of highly refined foods (flour, sugar, junk foods) and a water supply and soil deficient is chromium.

Get more chromium in meat, calf's liver, chicken, dairy, brewer's yeast, beer and whole grains, corn and corn oil, dried beans, brown rice, mushrooms and potatoes.

COPPER

Copper works in conjunction with zinc and vitamin C to form your skin's elastin. Associated with skin and hair coloring, copper is also associated with the sense of taste, involved in the healing process, energy production and essential for healthy nerves. Copper helps in forming hemoglobin and red blood cells. Essential for the connective tissue of the matrix, bone formation is among its many jobs, osteoporosis being an early sign of copper deficiency.

Sources include: plumbing (water pipes), cooking utensils, meats, organ meats (liver, kidney), salmon, seafood (lobster, shrimp, oysters), soybeans, nuts (pecans), beans, barley, oats, lentils, leafy greens, broccoli, beet roots, mushrooms, raisins, chocolate and blackstrap molasses.

High amounts of zinc or vitamin C reduce copper levels in the body, the reverse also being true. Long term use of copper cookware can cause an excess of copper.

GERMANIUM

An important trace mineral that works like hemoglobin. Germanium attaches itself to oxygen molecules, which are carried into the system *improving cellular oxygenation, oxygen being of prime immune importance in ridding the body of toxins.* A fast-acting painkiller, germanium, in a daily dose of 100–300 mg, can improve many illnesses, among which are: rheumatoid arthritis, food allergies, chronic viral infections, elevated cholesterol, candidiasis, cancer and AIDS.

Germanium is found in aloe vera, comfrey, garlic, ginseng, shitake mushrooms, onions and suma (herb).

IODINE

Important for healthy skin and thyroid function, but too much can result in acne. This trace mineral helps to metabolize excess fat. A lack of Iodine has been known to result in a goiter, recently however, a deficiency has been also linked to breast cancer.

Foods high in iodine include, iodized and sea salt, seafood, salt-water fish and seaweed (kelp, dulce), white deep-water fish, vegetables grown in iodine-rich soil (Southeastern US), garlic, limas, mushrooms, sesame seeds, soybeans, spinach (can also block, see below), summer squash, Swiss chard and turnip greens, whole wheat and peanuts.

When eaten raw in large amounts, the following block iodine uptake into the thyroid. They are: spinach, Brussels sprouts, cabbage, cauliflower, kale, peaches, pears, and turnips. If you have an underfunctioning thyroid, limit the above.

IRON

Vital for a fabu-lishous face, iron is instrumental in the formation of hemoglobin, which transports oxygen from the lungs to body tissues. This mineral, required for a healthy immune system, essential for energy and the production of many enzymes, is found in the largest amounts in the blood.

When taken with iron, vitamin C can increase absorption by 30 percent, but excessive amounts of zinc and vitamin E inhibit assimilation. Necessary for proper absorption are copper, manganese, molybdenum, vitamin A and the B-complex, as well as sufficient HCL (hydrochloric acid) in the stomach.

The utilization of iron is impaired by rheumatoid arthritis, and cancer; even with sufficient stores of iron in the liver, spleen and bone marrow, anemia will result, according to the

Journal of Orthomolecular Medicine. Iron is depleted by heavy exercise and perspiration, intestinal bleeding, heavy menstrual bleeding, excess phosphorus, ulcers, poor digestion, long-term or chronic illness, consumption of excess coffee or tea, prolonged use of antacids and any number of causes not linked to a nutritional deficiency. Sometimes a lack of B6 or B12 is the underlying problem. On the other hand, excessive iron in the body can cause the production of free-radicals.

Good iron sources include meat, liver, kidney, poultry, fish and seaweed (kelp, dulce), egg yolks, whole grains, enriched breads and cereals, lentils, millet, rice and wheat bran, limas and soybeans, sesame seeds, almonds, brewer's yeast, blackstrap molasses, radishes, beets, avocados, pumpkins, peaches, pears, raisins, dates and dried prunes.

MAGNESIUM

Important for the functioning of nerves, muscles, and an aid to the absorption of other minerals, including calcium and potassium, magnesium is vital to enzyme activity. Combined with vitamin B6 (pyridoxine), magnesium helps to dissolve calcium phosphate stones and may help to prevent calcium oxalate kidney stones.

Found in most foods, especially dairy, fish, meat and seafood, other magnesium-rich foods include apples, avocados, bananas, blackstrap molasses, brewer's yeast, whole grains, figs, garlic, kelp, limas, nuts and leafy greens.

Magnesium needs increase with the consumption of alcohol and diuretics and during spells of diarrhea. Magnesium absorption is inhibited by a high intake of fats, calcium, cod liver oil, vitamin D and protein, also foods high in oxalic acid. See *Calcium.*

MANGANESE

Essential for iron-deficiency anemia, minute amounts of manganese are needed for protein, purine and fat metabolism, healthy nerves and immune system function, and the regulation of blood sugar. Necessary for normal bone production and energy, manganese is also needed in order to utilize thiamine (B1). *Working with the entire B-complex, manganese gives an overall feeling of well-being.*

Best sources are nuts and seeds, avocados and whole grains, seaweed, blueberries, egg yolks, legumes, dried peas, pineapples, spinach and leafy greens.

MOLYBDENUM

Extremely small amounts are needed in nitrogen metabolism, yet a low intake is associated with cancer and mouth and gum disorders. Molybdenum helps to convert purines to uric acid, and promotes normal functioning of cells. Diets high in refined and processed foods may be deficient and a high intake of sulfur may also cause low levels. In older men, deficiency can cause sexual impotence. Exceedingly high daily intake (over 15 mg) may interfere with copper metabolism and may cause gout.

Good sources are beans, peas, legumes, cereal grains and leafy greens.

PHOSPHORUS

Needed for bone and tooth formation, cell growth, kidney function and contraction of the heart muscle, phosphorus helps convert food to energy and aids in the utilization of vitamins. It is rare to find a potassium deficiency. Found in most foods, particularly in sodas and junk foods, *concern is mainly to keep the necessary balance between magnesium, calcium and phosphorus.*

Most abundant in phosphorus are meat, poultry, fish and dairy products, eggs, bran and whole grains, seeds and nuts, legumes, dried fruit, brewer's yeast, garlic and asparagus.

POTASSIUM

Needed for a healthy nervous system, regular heart rhythm, and working with sodium to *maintain your body's water balance, potassium is important for cellular chemistry, regulating nutrient transfer to the cells.* Use of diuretics, laxatives, diarrhea, and kidney problems all upset potassium levels and the transmission of electrochemical impulses within the system. Needed for hormone secretion, stress-related hormones will decrease potassium-sodium levels within and outside of the cell.

Dietary sources of potassium include meat, poultry, fish, dairy products, whole grains, vegetables, legumes, nuts and fruit. Especially found in apricots, avocados, bananas, brewer's yeast and blackstrap molasses, brown rice, wheat bran, potatoes and yams, garlic, winter squash and dried fruit (raisins, dates, figs).

SELENIUM

This essential micro-nutrient, found in minute quantities in your body, *preserves the elasticity of your skin by protecting against free-radical damage.* A potent antioxidant, particularly when teamed with vitamin "E." A protector of the heart, immune system, pancreas and tissue elasticity. Deficiency is linked to cancer of the skin, prostate, colon, stomach, liver and breast. Hypertension, arteriosclerosis and heart disease have a definite vitamin E connection.

Dependent on soil content, selenium can be found in meat; chicken; seafood: tuna—packed in water, not oil—and salmon; dairy products, whole grains and wheat germ, Brazil nuts, blackstrap molasses, broccoli, garlic and onions. See also *Anti-Aging Antioxidants.*

SILICON (SILICA)

Very important for the connective tissue (collagen) in skin, hair and nails. Also needed for flexible arteries, silica plays a major part in cardiovascular disease. Necessary for the prevention of Alzheimer's disease, it counteracts the effects of aluminum deposits. Very important in the prevention of osteoporosis; with age, silicon levels drop necessitating larger dietary amounts for the elderly. Important for the proper utilization of silicon are minerals, boron, calcium, magnesium, manganese and potassium.

Good sources: alfalfa and whole grains, the herb horsetail, leafy greens, bell peppers, soybeans, beets and brown rice.

SODIUM

Necessary for *blood PH and water balance,* also, stomach, nerve and muscle function, sodium works with potassium. Rarely lacking, virtually all foods contain sodium; it is potassium that is usually deficient. Sodium deficiency, however, is noted by confusion, low blood sugar, weakness, dehydration, lethargy and heart palpitations. Excess results in edema, high blood pressure, potassium deficiency and possible, heart, liver, and/or kidney disease.

SULFUR

Super "skin"eral, anti-ager sulfur is needed for the maintenance of the elastic quality of the skin (elastin) and the synthesis of skin "glue" collagen. An acid-forming mineral, sulfur is part of the chemical structure of the longevity amino acids, methionine, cysteine, taurine and glutathione. Sulphur disinfects the blood, resists bacteria, guards cellular protoplasm, aids in oxidation reactions, stimulates liver bile secretion, while protecting against toxic substances, such as harmful effects of radiation and pollution.

Sulfur-containing foods include meat, eggs, fish, dried beans, soybeans, Brussels sprouts, kale and cabbage, turnips, garlic and onions, wheat germ and the herb horsetail; also, amino acids L-cysteine, L-lysine, L-cystine, and L-methionine. Sulfur can be purchased in tablet or powder form. See also *Anti-Aging Antioxidants.*

VANADIUM

Not easily absorbed, vanadium is *needed for cellular metabolism* and formation of teeth and bones. Inhibiting cholesterol synthesis, vanadium deficiency may be a link to cardiovascular and kidney disease. Low levels may also impair reproductive ability. A possible interaction may exist between vanadium and chromium. To be on the safe side, if you supplement, take them at different times.

Found in meat, fish, whole grains and vegetables oils, vanadium can also be obtained from radishes, dill, snap beans and olives.

ZINC

Important in skin metabolism, collagen production, protein synthesis and tissue repair, and necessary for a healthy immune system. Essential for prostate gland function and growth of the reproductive organs, as well as protecting the liver from chemical damage, sufficient intake and absorption of zinc is also needed to maintain vitamin E levels in the blood. Zinc

levels may drop because of diarrhea and fiber intake, the phy-
lates found in legumes and grains bind zinc so that it can't be
absorbed. Deficiencies may also result from consumption of
hard water, kidney disease, cirrhosis of the liver and diabetes.
More than 100 mg a day of supplemental zinc can impair the
immune system, under 100 mg can enhance response.

Good sources include meat, poultry, seafood, egg yolks,
milk, corn, hard cheese, nuts, peas, beans, wheat germ and
iron-rich foods.

ANTI-AGING
ANTIOXIDANTS

Antioxidants are a group of vitamins, minerals and enzymes that protect you from your own injured cells or particles cf cells called free-radicals. Missing part of their structure, your own cellular atoms or particles of cells try to link up with healthy cells. When they are successful, cross-linking occurs and your healthy cells become injured as well. Since all cells contain genetic material, the injured or cross-linked cells reproduce more injured cells. *Cross-linked cells show up on your skin as wrinkles, brown and white spots, cancerous and precancerous lesions and any number of little warts and blemishes, along with the sagging and deterioration associated with aging.*

With free-radical scavengers, or antioxidants roaming through your system, damaging free-radical cellular particles are neutralized protecting not only individual cells and your skin, but your entire immune system as well. Protected, you can resist infection and aging degenerative diseases which will also reflect in your complexion.

How are your cells injured in the first place? Free radicals can result from exposure to environmental pollution: radiation from TVs, microwaves, radio waves, cellular phones, computer terminals, bombardment from high tension wires and electrical appliances, and more—our environment is loaded with cellular threats; toxic chemicals in our environment—from pesticides and industrial wastes to auto exhaust; ultraviolet radiation from inadequate protection from the sun or suntanning beds; and the actions of our own body's metabolic processes, such as burning the stored fat molecules for energy.

There are three known free radicals: the superoxide, the hydroxyl and peroxide. In the normal course of events, damaged cells are kept in check by naturally occurring free radical "gobblers" that neutralize rampant cellular particles on site. Specific enzymes made naturally in the body are assigned the task. Four important ones are SOD (superoxide dismutase), catalase, methionine reductase, and glutathione peroxidase. These "gobblers" are aided by a diet rich in natural antioxidants and free radical scavengers, such as the vitamin A-C-Es, many of the B-complex vitamins, zinc, selenium, enzyme SOD (superoxide dismutase), the mineral selenium, essential fatty acid GLA (gamma-linoleic acid) and other nutrients.

Using antioxidants researchers have significantly extended the life of laboratory animals, as well as prevent, retard or postpone degenerative diseases such as cancer, and those diseases that are associated with aging, neutralizing destructive elements before they can harm healthy cellular membranes and rewrite your RNA/DNA, the genetic messages in your cells.

Antioxidants work together as synergies. To adequately protect your youthful glowing anti-aging skin and entire body, all the anti-agers must be available, along with water and all the other nutrients (vitamins, minerals, proteins, etc.) vital for your total well being. **They are all interrelated and depend on each other for proper assimilation.**

Most diets are lacking sufficient antioxidants and supporting nutrients to withstand the overwhelming amount of pollution we have to contend with today. Diets rich in the following nutrients and/or supplements that follow can beef up your anti-aging army. For supplemental information, see *Skin-Vites* and *"Skin" erals.*

VITAMIN A AND BETA CAROTENE

. . . promote germ-killing enzymes, destroy carcinogens (cancer-producing substances). Anti-agers and doctors using antioxidant nutrients as age-retarders use 15,000–35,000 IU of "A" and 25 mg beta carotene daily.

VITAMIN C

. . . increases interferon production, and powerfully stimulates T-effector cell (warrior cells sent by your thymus) activity along with being an exceedingly powerful antioxidant. Vitamin C reduces lipid production in the brain and spinal cord, frequent sites of free-radical damage. Significant amounts of "C" are needed to cross the blood-brain barrier. Bioflavonoids (particularly hesperidin) increase the potency of this anti-ager. Some anti-agers take megadoses of this vitamin, from 10–30 grams daily.

VITAMIN E

. . . a very powerful antioxidant that prevents the fats in the body and the cells from becoming rancid (lipid peroxidation). As far as we know it is the only antioxidant and free-radical scavenger whose major concern is to look after your body's lipid-based structures. (The more fat you eat, the more "E" you need.) Protecting the coating of each cell, "E" improves oxygenation and immune response.

A reminder that these anti-agers work synergistically, "E" needs zinc to maintain itself in normal blood concentrations, while allowing "A" to protect at a lower dosage. "E" also protects "C" and the B-complex from oxidation in the digestive tract, at the same time enhancing the activity of selenium and the amino acid cysteine.

Large doses of "E" have been shown to increase the life span of animals significantly. Animal experiments have shown that even low doses of vitamin E can protect lungs and tissues from damaging nitrous oxide and ozone in our atmosphere.

Most nutritionists agree that 400 mg of "E" daily is needed. An oil soluble vitamin that can temporarily elevate blood pressure, many physicians recommend doses of 100 mg to start working up to the optimum dosage. Many aging experts agree that a reasonable optimal daily intake is between 600–1200 mg daily. If you have a rheumatic heart, suffer from hypertension or a have a hyperthyroid **do not take high doses of supplemental "E."**

GAMMA-LINOLEIC ACID (GLA)

. . . an essential fatty acid that is the key regulator of the T-lymphocyte ("warrior cells," immune system protectors) function in the body. Linoleic acid found in cold pressed vegetable oils, plus zinc, magnesium, and Vitamins C, B6, B3, and A can be converted to GLA in the body. But if any of these are lacking the conversion is blocked. Other inhibitors include hydrogenated vegetable oils, margarine and high fatty diets. **Ready-made GLA is found in evening primrose oil, black currant seed oil and borage oil.** See also *A Splash of Oil*.

L-CYSTEINE

. . . a powerful detoxifier of alcohol, tobacco smoke and environmental pollutants, is used by the liver and the lymphocytes to detoxify environmental pollutants, chemicals and germ poisons. A sulphur-containing amino acid, it is needed to produce glutathione. One of the best free-radical "gobblers," it functions best when taken with selenium and vitamin E. Supplementation is often recommended for rheumatoid arthritis. This toxic metal remover has a chelating effect, removing excess copper from the body. It also promotes muscle building and the burning of fat. Due to its ability to break down mucous in the respiratory tract, it is of benefit in treating bronchitis, emphysema and TB (tuberculosis). Very unstable, cysteine easily converts to L-cystine; as supplements each will be equally beneficial. Anti-agers recommend 500–1500 mg daily taken on an empty stomach ½ hour before meal or before bedtime.

L-GLUTATHIONE

. . . another powerful antioxidant, protecting from degenerating drugs, alcohol and tobacco smoke. Detoxifying the body of metals, the amino acid helps in treating blood and liver disorders, also helps to diminish the side effects of X-rays and chemotherapy. Longevity dosage same as above.

SELENIUM

. . . a very exciting anti-cancer, anti-aging micro-nutrient, that preserves the elasticity of your skin by inhibiting oxidation of polyunsaturated fatty acids and the resultant cross-linking of proteins. Working synergistically with its partner vitamin E, selenium is essential for the "germ warfare" stimulator, key enzyme, glutathione peroxidase, mentioned earlier. Selenium, alone, seems to be the most effective antioxidant for those who are sensitive to chemicals in the environment. Clinical ecologists have reported that 400 mcg supplemental selenium daily can clear up symptoms in about 60 percent of chemical allergy sufferers. Works synergistically with the vitamin "ACEs."

SOD (SUPEROXIDE DISMUTASE)

... an enzyme produced in the body along with its partner catalase. Part of your system's first line of defense against unstable oxygen species and free radicals, it is found in all cells. Protection against the damaging effects of oxygen is its primary function. SOD levels in your body seem to be directly proportional to your life span and closely tied to aging. Healthy bodies produce nearly 5 million units of SOD daily, and while free-radical production increases with aging, SOD levels drop. Given by injection, SOD has shown remarkable healing effects, reversing degeneration. It reduced inflammation, alleviated the pain of arthritis, lessened or prevented the side effects of high radiation doses, and may possibly prevent the growth of cancer cells. Oral supplementation with SOD, however, is controversial, since it is a long chain protein which biochemists believe cannot cross the cell membrane.

Foods containing SOD include barley grass, wheat grass, broccoli, Brussels sprouts and cabbage and most green plants.

See *Skin-Vites* and *"Skin" erals* for further information.

VI.
RECAPPING AND
RESOURCES

SKIN CARE ROUTINES

MORNING CLEANSING

1. Splash face with warm water.
2. Apply cold pressed oil (with balancing essential oils, if possible) with upward and outward light massaging strokes.
3. *Options:*
   A great time for the freeze lift.
   Or . . . Cleansing with a light exfoliant.
4. Rinse thoroughly with warm water.
5. Tone.
6. Apply your day cream, lotion, moisturizer or intensive care oils.

EVENING CLEANSING

1. Remove all makeup with light cold pressed oil and moistened cotton pads.
2. Apply a little more oil and lightly massage face and neck using upward and outward strokes.
3. Deep cleanse using a *fruity peel* or *mechanical exfoliant.*
4. Tone.
5. Apply nightly marinade or intensive healing treatment.

STEPS FOR FREEZE LIFT

1. Splash face with warm water
2. If deep cleansing, cleanse; rinse. Pat dry. For dry, sensitive or mature skin, a light oil cleansing is sufficient in the morning, provided, of course, all makeup was removed and the face cleansed the night before.
3. Apply a good solid weight cold pressed oil or heavy cream as a base for cleansing. I use extra virgin olive oil with essential oil of Lavender, Geranium, and/or Fennel.
4. Proceed with the freeze lift by splashing your cheeks and neck with ice cube water until it is numb, and icy.
5. When finished pat dry and add a dab of moisturizer, your day dressing or intensive oil. A toner isn't necessary since pores are already tightened, skin is perky and your day dressing is nutritious.

STEPS FOR FACIAL

Option #1. Using a Facial Scrub or Mask and Scented Massage.

1. Cleanse as usual, removing all makeup (a light oil cleansing will do).
2. Apply scented oil and massage, leave on face 15 minutes.
3. Facial Steam or sauna. Nothing more than a warm compress for Sensitive skin, or skin with broken capillaries.
4. Facial Scrub (not for broken caps) or Facial mask with thorough rinsing.
5. Apply toner.
6. Moisturize with day or night dressing or intensive healing oils.

Wait for at least for at least 20 minutes to apply makeup. Longer, if possible.

Option #2. Using the Facial Scrub without the scented massage. Proceed as above, omitting step 2.

Option #3. Scented oil massage and acid or enzyme *Fruity Peel* exfoliant.

1. Cleanse, removing all makeup.
2. Apply scented oil and massage, leave on face 15 minutes.
3. Remove excess oil.
4. Apply "Fruity Peel."
5. Steam or apply compress.
6. Rinse.
7. Tone.
8. Moisturize with day or night dressing, or intensive care treatment.

Do not apply makeup for at least 20 minutes.

Option #4. Fruity Peel without the scented massage. Proceed as above omitting steps 2 and 3.

See *Fruity Peels*.

SELECTED BIBLIOGRAPHY

Andrecht, Venus Catherine. *The Herb Lady's Notebook*. Ramona, CA: Ransom Hill Press, 1988.

Balch, James F. and Phyllis A. Balch. *Prescription for Nutritional Healing*. Garden City Park, NY: Avery Publishing Group, Inc., 1990.

Bihova, Diana and Connie Schrader. *Beauty from the Inside Out*. New York: Rawson Associates, 1987.

Bricklin, Mark, ed. *The Practical Encyclopedia of Natural Healing*. Emmaus, PA: Rodale Press, Inc., 1976.

Brumberg, Elaine. *Take Care of Your Skin*. New York: Harper and Row, 1989.

Castleton, Virginia. *Secrets of Natural Beauty*. New Canaan, CT: Keats Publishing, Inc. 1978.

Chaitow, Leon. *Amino Acids in Therapy: A Guide to Therapeutic Application of Protein Constituents*. Rochester, VT: Healing Arts Press, 1988.

Clark, Linda. *Secrets of Health and Beauty*. New York: Pyramid, 1976.

Chase, Deborah. *The New Medically Based No-Nonsense Beauty Book*. New York: Henry Holt and Company, 1989.

Clayman, Charles B., ed. *The American Medical Association Home Medical Encyclopedia*. New York: Random House, 1989.

Davis, Patricia. *Aromatherapy A-Z*. Saffron Walden, U.K.: The C.W. Daniel Co., Ltd., 1988.

Erdmann, Robert with Meirion Jones. *The Amino Revolution*. New York: Contemporary Books, Inc. 1987.

Feder, Lewis M. and Jane MacLean Craig. *About Face*. New York: Warner Books, 1989.

Frank, Benjamin S. with Philip Miele. *Dr. Frank's No Aging Diet*. New York: Dial Press, 1976.

Grieve, M. A Modern Herbal. *The Medical, Culinary, Cosmetic and Economic Properties, Cultivation and Folk-Lore of Herbs, Grasses, Fungi Shrubs & Trees with all Their Modern Scientific Uses* (two vols.). New York: Dover, 1982.

Hendriksen, Ole. *Ole Hendriksen's Seven-Day Skin-Care Program: The*

Scandinavian Method for a Radiant Complexion. New York: Macmillan, 1984.

Kenton, Leslie. *Ageless Aging: The Natural Way to Stay Young*. New York: Grove Press, Inc., 1986.

Kirschman, John D. with Lavon J. Dunn. *Nutrition Almanac*. New York: McGraw-Hill, 1984.

Krane, Jessica. *How to Use Your Hands to Save Your Face: Faceometrics*. New York: Avon, 1969.

Lust, John. *The Herb Book*. New York: Bantam, 1987.

Nachtigall, Lila and Joan Rattner Heilman. *Estrogen: The Facts Can Save Your Life*. Los Angeles: The Body Press, 1986.

Newman, Laura. *Make Your Juicer Your Drug Store*. New York: Benedict Lust Publications, 1970.

Mindell, Earl. *Earl Mindell's New and Revised Vitamin Bible: How the Right Vitamins and Nutrient Supplements Can Help Turn Your Life Around*. New York: Warner Books, 1985.

Price, Shirley. *Practical Aromatherapy: How to Use Essential Oils to Restore Vitality*. London: Thorsons, 1987.

Quinlin, Patrick. *Healing Nutrients: The People's Guide to Using Common Nutrients That Will Help You Feel Better Than You Ever Thought Possible*. New York: Contemporary Books. 1987.

Rose, Jeanne. *Jeanne Rose's Herbal*. New York: Perigee, 1983.

———. *Jeanne Rose's Herbal Body Book*. New York: Perigee, 1976.

Soltanoff, Jack. *Natural Healing: The Total Health and Nutrition Program That Helps You Keep Your Body Disease-Free Every Day of Your Life*. New York: Warner Books, 1988.

Tenny, Louise. *Today's Herbal Health*. Provo, UT: Woodland Books, 1983.

Tisserand, Robert B. *The Art of Aromatherapy: The Healing and Beautifying Properties of the Essential Oils of Flowers and Herbs*. Rochester, VT: Healing Arts Press, 1977.

Tisserand, Maggie. *Aromatherapy for Women: A Practical Guide to Essential Oils for Health and Beauty*. Rochester, VT: Healing Arts Press, 1988.

Walker, N. W. *Raw Vegetable Juices*. New York: Pyramid Books, 1975.

Wesley-Hosford, Zia. *Face Value: Skin Care for Women Over 35*. New York: Bantam, 1986.

ESSENTIAL OILS

Resources

   Aroma Vera Inc. 310–280–0407. 5901 Rodeo Road, Los Angeles, CA 90016.

   Body Naturals/OSA East Coast. 516–351–6166. 333 New York Ave., Huntington, NY 11743.

   Essential Imports. 619–471–8765. P.O. Box 53, Cardiff, CA 92007–0053.

   Esthetique. 800–446–2260. 580 Lancaster Avenue. Bryn Mawr, PA 19010.

   Ledet Oils. 916–965–7546. 4611 Awani Court, Fair Oaks, CA 95628.

   Lifetree Aromatix. 818–986–0594. 3949 Longridge Ave. Sherman Oaks, CA 91423. *Information package $2.50.*

   OSA. 415–459–3998. P.O. Box 6482 *or* 28 Paul Drive, Suite F, San Rafael, CA 94903.

   Time Laboratories. 818–300–8096. P.O. Box 3243, South Pasadena, CA 91031.

   Windrose Aromatics Inc. 602–861–3696. 12629 N. Tatum Blvd. Suite 611, Phoenix, AZ 85032.

For more information: **Contact ASPA—The American Assn. for Phytotherapy and Aromatherapy International. 818–457–1742. Fax. 818–300–8099.** P.O. Box 3679, South Pasadena, CA 91031.

INDEX

ABOUT THE AUTHOR

Julia Busch researches *beauty* in its broadest sense. A life-long health and well-being enthusiast, she has written on a wide variety of topics, from TMJ, temporomandibular (jaw) joint, problems to facial massage techniques, to the "aging in a youth society dilemma," most recently contributing to *Let's Live* and *InnerSelf* magazines.

Her first book was released in the early 1970s. Ms. Busch has a certificate in aromatherapy, publishes the Anti-Aging Press and co-hosts "Youthfully Yours" on Talk America. Sharing the information she garners in the area of holistic care and "youth extension," Julia's first anti-aging offering, *Facelift Naturally, The At-Home or Anywhere, Painless, Natural Facelift for Men and Women That Really Works!* lifts the face, while energizing the body.

Writing for all ages, she lifts the spirit in *Positively Young!* erasing "wrinkles on the *inside*" with "youth games," "self-love games," laugh lessons and stress releasing games for the nineties. Her audio cassette, *Youth and Skin Secrets Revealed,* encompasses a wide variety of holistic topics.

Julia's diverse background includes the study of voice and opera at Juilliard School of Music; sculpture and art history at Columbia and the University of Miami (where she also taught drawing and composition); and teaching humanities at Miami Dade Community College. She authored *A Decade of Sculpture: The Media of the 1960s;* has written for the *Art Journal* and *Ideas* magazine; and designed women's clothing and fine jewelry while researching plastic as an art form and contributing to books on the same subject.

Julia believes in living, loving, laughing, maintaining a dream, a youthful spirit and a holistic life-style—*this book is a perfect example!*

KEEP TRACK OF YOUR DIET
–AND YOUR HEALTH!

__ THE SODIUM COUNTER   0-425-08779-4/$3.50
WILLIAM I. KAUFMAN
High blood pressure has been linked to many
of the deaths in the United States–and high
consumption of salt has been proven to aggravate
this dangerous condition. Here are ways to cut
down on unnecessary salt in your diet.

WILLIAM I. KAUFMAN'S
WATCH-YOUR-DIET SERIES
Extra-small and slender guides to carry with
you everywhere you shop and eat!

__CALORIE COUNTER FOR 6 QUICK-LOSS DIETS
  0-515-10406-4/$3.50
__CALORIE GUIDE TO BRAND NAMES
  0-515-10559-7/$2.95
__CHOLESTEROL CONTROL GRAM COUNTER
  0-515-10562-7/$2.95
__THE NEW LOW CARBOHYDRATE DIET
  0-515-10563-5/$3.50

Payable in U.S. funds. No cash orders accepted. Postage & handling: $1.75 for one book, 75¢
for each additional. Maximum postage $5.50. Prices, postage and handling charges may
change without notice. Visa, Amex, MasterCard call 1-800-788-6262, ext. 1, refer to ad # 242

Or, check above books   Bill my: ☐ Visa   ☐ MasterCard   ☐ Amex
and send this order form to: (expires)
The Berkley Publishing Group   Card#_____
390 Murray Hill Pkwy., Dept. B   ($15 minimum)
East Rutherford, NJ 07073   Signature_____
Please allow 6 weeks for delivery.   Or enclosed is my: ☐ check   ☐ money order

Name_____   Book Total $_____

Address_____   Postage & Handling $_____

City_____   Applicable Sales Tax $_____
                                         (NY, NJ, PA, CA, GST Can.)
State/ZIP_____   Total Amount Due $_____

ENHANCE FAMILY LIFE

__MOMMY THERE'S NOTHING TO DO
  Cynthia MacGregor   0-425-13911-5/$4.50
A collection of easy ideas children can enjoy with
parents or alone on rainy days, long trips, or any time.

*Don't miss these Cynthia MacGregor
titles for even more family entertainment...*

__FREE FAMILY FUN   0-425-14367-8/$4.50
__TOTALLY TERRIFIC FAMILY GAMES
                         0-425-14574-3/$4.99

__THE HOMEWORK PLAN
  Linda Sonna, Ph.D.   0-425-14499-2/$4.99
**"A homework survival handbook for busy
parents..."**—*Positive Parenting* magazine
Education expert and psychologist Linda Sonna
reveals simple methods to enrich communication
and improve your child's performance.

__STRESS STRATEGIES FOR PARENTS
  Kimberly Barrett, Ph.D.   0-425-13626-4/$4.99
Dr. Barrett offers busy parents smart strategies to help
them handle stress...and handle their children with the
right mix of attention, discipline and love.

Payable in U.S. funds. No cash orders accepted. Postage & handling: $1.75 for one book, 75¢
for each additional. Maximum postage $5.50. Prices, postage and handling charges may
change without notice. Visa, Amex, MasterCard call 1-800-788-6262, ext. 1, refer to ad # 537

Or, check above books	Bill my: ☐ Visa ☐ MasterCard ☐ Amex	
and send this order form to:		(expires)
The Berkley Publishing Group	Card#	
390 Murray Hill Pkwy., Dept. B		($15 minimum)
East Rutherford, NJ 07073	Signature	
Please allow 6 weeks for delivery.	Or enclosed is my: ☐ check ☐ money order	
Name	Book Total	$
Address	Postage & Handling	$
City	Applicable Sales Tax $	
	(NY, NJ, PA, CA, GST Can.)	
State/ZIP	Total Amount Due	$

**THE COMPLETE GUIDE ALL PARENTS
SHOULD HAVE WHEN TRAVELING**

THE FAMILY VACATION HEALTH AND SAFETY GUIDE

Linda R. Bernstein, Pharm. D.

A comprehensive handbook with advice on:

*Packing and Preparing
First Aid
Traveling Safely in Foreign Countries
Traveling with Children and Pets
Dealing with Illness Away from Home*

This convenient reference addresses the kinds of emergencies families can experience while traveling. It prepares parents for simple injuries, such as rashes and sunburn; and advises on important issues, like Red Cross procedures for emergency aid and special precautions for foreign countries.

__0-425-14297-3/$4.99   *(Coming in June)*

Payable in U.S. funds. No cash orders accepted. Postage & handling: $1.75 for one book, 75¢ for each additional. Maximum postage $5.50. Prices, postage and handling charges may change without notice. Visa, Amex, MasterCard call 1-800-788-6262, ext. 1, refer to ad # 538

Or, check above books Bill my: ☐ Visa ☐ MasterCard ☐ Amex	
and send this order form to:	(expires)
The Berkley Publishing Group	Card#_____
390 Murray Hill Pkwy., Dept. B	($15 minimum)
East Rutherford, NJ 07073	Signature_____
Please allow 6 weeks for delivery.	Or enclosed is my: ☐ check ☐ money order
Name_____	Book Total $_____
Address_____	Postage & Handling $_____
City_____	Applicable Sales Tax $_____ (NY, NJ, PA, CA, GST Can.)
State/ZIP_____	Total Amount Due $_____